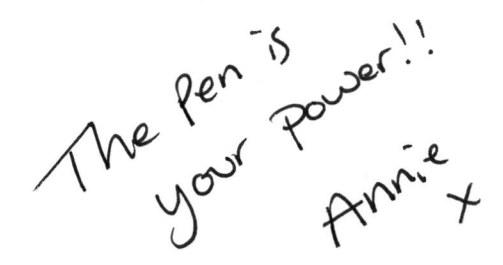

ANNIE HUMPHRIS

The Maternal Mindset

A journal for all mums going through the postnatal journey

The Pen is your Power!!
Annie x

AUSTIN MACAULEY PUBLISHERS™
LONDON • CAMBRIDGE • NEW YORK • SHARJAH

Copyright © Annie Humphris 2024

The right of Annie Humphris to be identified as author of this work has been asserted by the author in accordance with sections 77 and 78 of the Copyright, Designs and Patents Act 1988.

All rights reserved. No part of this publication may be reproduced, stored in a retrieval system, or transmitted in any form or by any means, electronic, mechanical, photocopying, recording, or otherwise, without the prior permission of the publishers.

Any person who commits any unauthorised act in relation to this publication may be liable to criminal prosecution and civil claims for damages.

The information in this book has been put together by way of providing general guidance in relation to the specific subjects addressed. It is not meant to be relied upon or used as a substitute for any medical, healthcare or any other professional advice or treatment. It is imperative that the user consults a medical professional such as a doctor before you change, stop or start any medical treatment. The author will not be liable for loss, harm or damage arising from any information or suggestion within this book.

The author is aware that all of the information given and complied in this book is correct and up to date at the time of publication. The author does not assume any responsibility for errors or changes that take place after publication has happened.

A CIP catalogue record for this title is available from the British Library.

ISBN 9781035855896 (Paperback)
ISBN 9781035855902 (Hardback)
ISBN 9781035855919 (ePub e-book)

www.austinmacauley.com

First Published 2024
Austin Macauley Publishers Ltd®
1 Canada Square
Canary Wharf
London
E14 5AA

ACKNOWLEDGEMENTS

A huge thank you to the incredible mums who contributed to this book: baring your soul to the world is no easy task. Your strength as mothers is inspirational; you are all guiding lights, who are so truly kind and wonderful. Thank you for helping me make this journal a reality.

To my wonderful husband: you are the love of my life, and I am so grateful for all of your help and unjudgemental love in supporting me through the dark and light times. You are one of the most selfless people on this planet and always support me in achieving my goals. You have been instrumental in helping me create this journal and have given me so much confidence to do so – from the bottom of my heart, thank you.

My girl gang deserve a special shout out! Their support, knowledge and guidance has not only made me the mother that I am today but they too helped me create, design and curate this journal. My true soul sisters, who I am thankful for every day, thank you for always championing me to be the best I can be in every single aspect of my life and for all of your help. I would be lost without you all and am so thankful for all of your help and love.

A huge thank you to Emma, who helped me create the pages dedicated to children with additional needs. You are a truly spectacular mother who hasn't had a smooth road, but you have done it with such grace. You are a very strong and inspirational person.

To my wonderful friends, family and sister who so patiently helped me create this, and listened to me as I bounced ideas back and forth – you are all incredible and you all helped me make this a safe place for all to write their hopes, dreams, fears and more. Your support has been invaluable; you all inspire me to be the best I can be each and every day. I would be lost without you all and your love.

AUTHOR'S NOTE

This book is intended for all of those mums who need a safe space to pour their heart out without judgement, to write down their feelings and to let out all of the love, pain, worries and joy they feel throughout their motherhood journey after birth. I feel so passionately that not enough people talk about the hardships of parenting or even how they got there; it seems as though everyone bottles everything up. So, I wanted to give people a safe space to come to terms with their parenting journey.

After the birth of my son Quinton, I struggled massively with not feeling like I was enough. I just didn't feel like I had done enough and that I deserved this perfect precious miracle. I truly didn't feel that I was a good enough mother for him and that he would be better off without me. I wasn't a good enough friend, sister, daughter or wife. I felt like no one could hear me or see me. I felt as though I had to be grateful and always happy in front of people – but I was screaming inside. I felt I had no right to feel like I did because of the journey we had to get him in the first place. The pressure was intolerable: my self-esteem was at an all-time low, and I just didn't know how to navigate all of these overwhelming feelings. One day, I just screamed and sobbed with physical and mental exhaustion whilst my husband held me on the kitchen floor. I sought help from a medical professional who told me it was just my hormones from my PCOS (polycystic ovary syndrome) and it would settle down with exercise and eating right. Anyone who knows me would be aware that I follow a good diet, take the right supplements, and exercise a lot in order to keep myself 'balanced'. I had never felt so alone, unheard and unseen; I knew it was more than my hormones. So I took to journalling – something that helped me in the past during low periods. Gradually, with the help of the journal, my amazing husband, family and the most incredible set of girlfriends, I came to terms with the last few years and how to accept my new life with a baby, my new body and how to find a 'new normal'. I have learnt that I am enough, that all I did brought us our boy, that I am now stronger and more confident than ever and can fully appreciate our perfect boy..

Creating this journal has been amazing. I have learnt so much about myself, but most importantly I have learnt so much about the wonderful women who contributed to it – many of whom suffered in silence, out of fear of judgement and not knowing how opening up would be received. Reading many of these anecdotes about how much these mums struggled and still are struggling, my heart broke. I want to try to remove the stigma of struggling alone as a mum and I hope to give people the confidence to not only own their feelings but to grow and flourish from them and their journey through motherhood.

So few people talk about fertility or infertility, miscarriage, birth and how hard the recovery is after birth. I was not prepared for how horrendous the post-birth recovery is and how you are expected just to 'bounce back' and get on with your daily life straight away. You are suddenly in charge of keeping a human alive, all whilst you recover physically and mentally yourself – it is one hell of a task. No matter how prepared you are, you are thrown into motherhood, and most mothers are expected to shoulder the burden alone as it's 'a mother's job and the dad helps out'. In reality, it took two people to make this life. Raising a child takes a village, and no one should have to carry this responsibility alone.

As a mum you so often lose yourself and lose your identity. There is so much pressure on mums these days that you are criticised if you are a working mum or a stay-at-home mum, if you breastfeed or not, if you feed your child pre-brought snacks or not. In every baby class, someone always seems to be watching with prying eyes as you change a nappy, if you let them cry or not, how you feed or discipline them and even how you hold your baby. All this comparison and judgement is all consuming and exhausting – it is no wonder that mothers feel the pressure and feelings that they do. I felt and still feel in many ways like I am consistently second-guessing myself. So, after much deliberation and a nagging feeling of wanting to help any mums who feel they are suffering alone because they don't want to feel more judgment or don't feel ready to open up, The 'Maternal Mindset Journal' was born. In this journal there is no judgement. I wanted the user to find out who they want to be, to reclaim their identity, self-love, and live their life as they want to.

Motherhood is a journey, it isn't a race.

Annie
X

CONTENTS

Introduction 9

My Birth Story 10

About My Baby 16

Milestones 18

Changing Bag Check List 20

What you can include in your Daily Journal 22

'You Time' Ideas 56

You Time Ideas from 'Real Life Mums' 57

Handling Overwhelm 60

Mum Hacks 98

Signs of Postnatal Depression/Anxiety and How to Seek Help 135

'Real Life Mums' Who Knew They Needed Help When... 137

Managing Mum Burnout 209

Expectations vs Reality 245

Affirmations 281

Advice from 'Real Life Mums' 317

Identity and How to Find Yourself Again 355

Bobby's Story 391

Signs Your Child Could Have Additional Challenges 397

What to do if Your Child is Showing Signs of having Additional
    Challenges 398

Positive Attributes You Want to Pass on to Your Child 433

Funny Stories from 'Real Life Mums' 469

Film & Boxset Recommendations 506

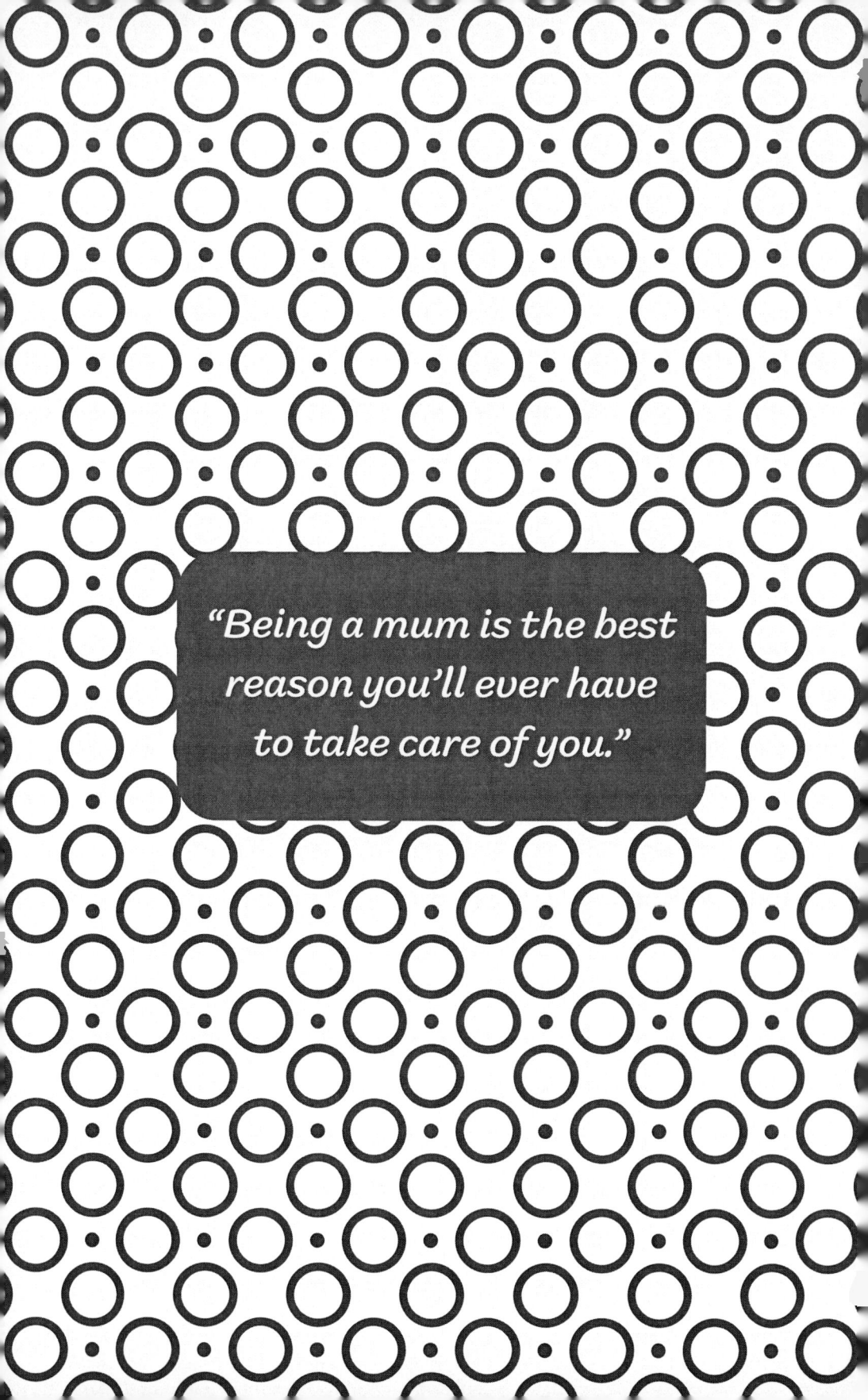

"Being a mum is the best reason you'll ever have to take care of you."

INTRODUCTION

Becoming a mum is the happiest, hardest, worst, best, easiest and most stressful stress-free journey you will ever go on. No matter how long it took you to get you to the point of the arrival of your little person, and no matter how many speed-bumps you encountered to get there, it is a roller-coaster of emotions. With trying to conceive, fertility and infertility obstacles, miscarriage and waiting for them to arrive, there is always a tidal wave of emotions that are mixed with good and bad life changes to come to terms with. Everything as a mum is magnified. There is so much advice online and in books, it's hard to know what to follow – one size doesn't fit all, and it's okay to pull from a range of parenting techniques or create your own. I truly believe that this culture of telling you how to parent needs to stop. I want this journal to give the user back the power to find and carve their own path.

This journal was created to give you a safe space to get those feelings out of your mind and on to paper. The good, the bad and the ugly. There are a few handy tips, tricks, hacks and check lists within the book, along with some wonderful anecdotes from 'Real Life Mums'. On the whole I have tried my best to make it simple to read so not to overwhelm you with information and lots of words, boxes or graphics that you might not have the time or brain space to read and digest.

Its main aim is to create a safe space for both new and experienced mums who might be having their next little one, to cathartically release their thoughts with no judgement.

MY BIRTH STORY

Writing down your birth story can be an incredibly cathartic way of digesting and accepting what you went through – whether it was a good or difficult birth. More often than not, births do not go to plan and everyone's birth is always different. It is an important part of recovery and a wonderful record to have written down.

> How to record your birth story:
> - How did you feel when the birth started and also during labour?
> - What were your main worries?
> - Did you have pain relief? Did it differ from your plan?
> - Did your birth go as you had hoped and planned?
> - How did you feel when you met baby for the first time?
> - Did you have to stay in hospital? What was that like, and how did it make you feel?
> - How did you feel when you left hospital?
> - How did you feel when you got home?
> - How did your birth partner feel and help you during and after labour?

_____
_____
_____
_____
_____
_____

MY BIRTH STORY

MY BIRTH STORY

"There is no such thing as being a perfect parent."

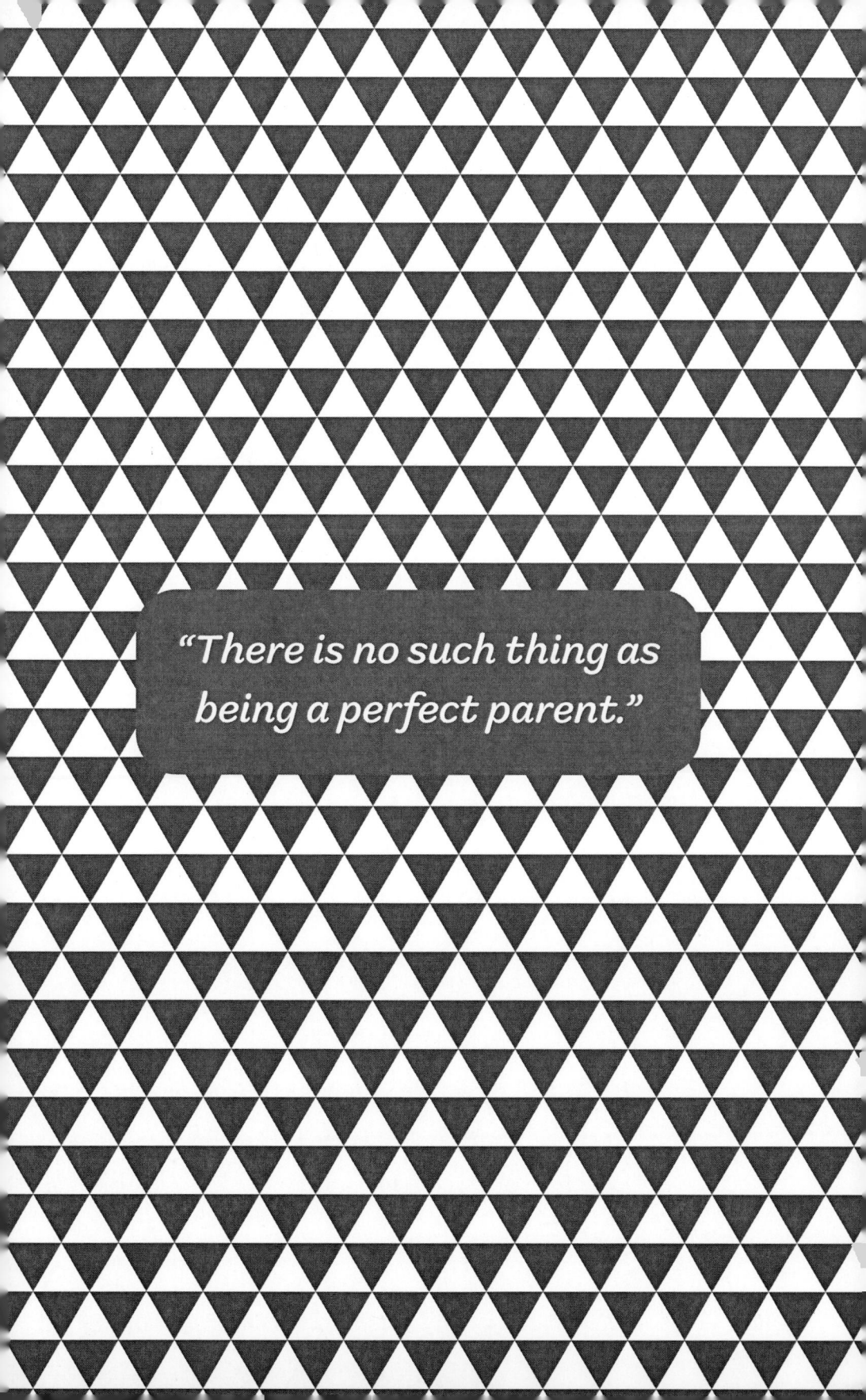

ABOUT MY BABY

- Name: _____
- Date of birth: _____
- Time of birth: _____
- Duration of labour: _____
- Where baby was born: _____
- Weather during labour: _____
- Weight: _____
- Length: _____
- Eye colour: _____
- Hair colour: _____
- First visitors: _____
- News headlines: _____
- Head of state: _____
- Price of milk: _____
- Price of postage: _____
- Price of petrol: _____
- Shared birthdays: _____

Notes:

_____
_____
_____
_____
_____
_____
_____

ABOUT MY BABY

MILESTONES

- First smile: _____
- First laugh: _____
- Baby recognised you: _____
- Held head up: _____
- Sat: _____
- Rolled over: _____
- Crawled: _____
- Food: _____
- Slept through the night: _____
- Tooth: _____
- Word: _____
- Steps: _____
- Your first date night: _____
- Night out with loved ones: _____
- Family holiday: _____
- Your first alcoholic drink: _____
- First meal at home post labour: _____
- Mum & baby first solo outing: _____
- First post baby sex: _____

Other milestones that you have celebrated:

_____
_____
_____
_____
_____

CHANGING BAG CHECK LIST

- Nappies and nappy bags
- Wipes
- Breast pads
- Barrier cream
- Change of clothes and hat for baby
- Change of top, clothes or scarf for you (it helps with any accidents!!)
- Changing mat
- Snacks for you or your little one (depending on age)
- Baby first aid kit
- Comforter and/or small toys
- Antibacterial wipes or spray
- Water for you and your little one (depending on age)
- Muslin squares
- A dirty clothes bag (a freezer bag works great!)
- Baby sunscreen
- Teething gel
- Dummies – if you are using them
- Bibs, spoons, reusable place mat and food (if you are weaning)
- Nipple shields and nipple cream (if breastfeeding)
- Any medicines you or baby might need
- Nursing cover
- Bottle warmer or flask of boiled water

Notes:

WHAT YOU CAN INCLUDE IN YOUR DAILY JOURNAL

- What is upsetting or worrying you in that moment?
- Parenting worries or troubles.
- Things you want to change or improve.
- What you are grateful for?
- What is overwhelming you?
- Record your good or bad dreams or any flashbacks you could be having.
- Burnout: why you are feeling it and how you can feel better?
- Long-term visions of where you want to be.
- Reflections or revelations.
- What you are grateful for?
- Exciting firsts you or your baby have achieved.
- What you are enjoying about parenting or what you aren't enjoying.
- Feelings you have at that moment in time.
- Recording big life events.
- Worries or struggles you are having with your little one.
- Relationship struggles.
- Frustrations that you might have.
- Ending with an affirmation can be a really positive ending to a good or tough day.
- Things you have achieved in that day or hope to achieve that week.

Notes:

WHAT YOU CAN INCLUDE IN YOUR DAILY JOURNAL

Daily Journal

Date: _____

Daily Journal

Date: _____

Daily Journal

Date: _____

JOURNAL: WEEK ONE

Daily Journal

Date: _____

Daily Journal

Date: _____

Daily Journal

Date: _____

Daily Journal

Date: _____

Weekly Check-In

Date: _____

Top 3 things I did this week:

_____

_____

_____

This week I felt:

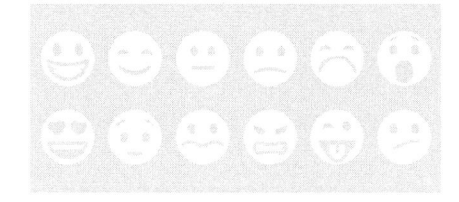

Milestones:

Next week I would like to:

_____

_____

_____

Things I am proud of this week:

Things to celebrate:

Things to let go of:

My ranking of the week:

☆ ☆ ☆ ☆ ☆

JOURNAL: WEEK ONE

Daily Journal

Date: _____

Daily Journal

Date: _____

Daily Journal Date: _____

Daily Journal

Date: _____

Daily Journal

Date: _____

JOURNAL: WEEK TWO

Daily Journal

Date: _____

Daily Journal Date: _____

Weekly Check-In

Date: _____

Top 3 things I did this week:

_____

_____

_____

Milestones:

This week I felt:

Next week I would like to:

_____

_____

_____

Things I am proud of this week:

Things to celebrate:

Things to let go of:

My ranking of the week:

☆ ☆ ☆ ☆ ☆

JOURNAL: WEEK TWO

Daily Journal

Date: _____

Daily Journal

Date: _____

Daily Journal

Date: _____

Daily Journal

Date: _____

Daily Journal

Date: _____

JOURNAL: WEEK THREE

Daily Journal

Date: _____

Daily Journal

Date: _____

Weekly Check-In

Date: _____

Top 3 things I did this week:

_____

_____

_____

This week I felt:

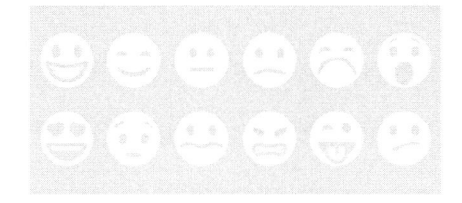

Milestones:

Next week I would like to:

_____

_____

_____

Things I am proud of this week:

Things to celebrate:

Things to let go of:

My ranking of the week:

☆ ☆ ☆ ☆ ☆

JOURNAL: WEEK THREE

Daily Journal

Date: _____

Daily Journal

Date: _____

Daily Journal

Date: _____

Daily Journal

Date: _____

Daily Journal

Date: _____

JOURNAL: WEEK FOUR

Daily Journal

Date: _____

Daily Journal

Date: _____

Weekly Check-In

Date: _____

Top 3 things I did this week:

_____

_____

_____

This week I felt:

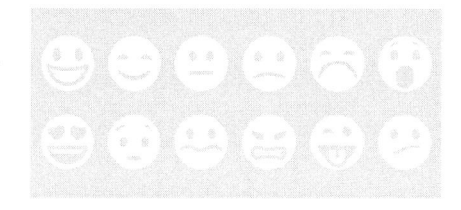

Milestones:

Next week I would like to:

_____

_____

_____

Things I am proud of this week:

Things to celebrate:

Things to let go of:

My ranking of the week:

☆ ☆ ☆ ☆ ☆

JOURNAL: WEEK FOUR   55

'YOU TIME' IDEAS

Allowing yourself to have your own time is vital to restoring yourself, no matter the age of your child. Finding just a snippet of time in a day will make a huge difference to your mental state and well-being. It is okay to have non-negotiable 'you time'; remember, a happy mum makes for happy children. Showing your children what lights you up and what breathes fire back into your soul is a fantastic way to help them grow and develop as well-rounded people. Take some 'you time' and don't feel guilty for it!

Go for a walk

·

Take a long bath

·

Have a pamper with a face or foot mask

·

Meditate

·

Watch one of your favourite shows

·

Listen to a podcast or audiobook

·

Go out and enjoy a beauty treatment

·

Take a nap

·

Do a light workout or yoga

·

Go and have your hair done

·

Enjoy your favourite hobby

·

Meet a friend for a catch-up

·

Book a night out with friends

YOU TIME IDEAS FROM 'REAL LIFE MUMS'

On a Saturday or Sunday my husband takes our girls out for a few hours, so that I can have a pamper and a long bath – to feel more like me.

Vikki – Mum of Jessica (2) and Emillia (3 months)

✸ ✸ ✸

I make sure since having Finley I maintain a level of my 'old' life. I continue to regularly go to the gym three to four times a week, see friends in the evenings, have massages and even go away for long weekends with the girls. How do I do this?... The practical answer is – my husband. We have a shared calendar and have the agreement that if the day or night is free we can book things in with our friends/have our alone time. (Of course, this is within reason, and we make sure we have a good balance of family life as well as friends time.) I made a promise to myself to maintain my friendship groups and see my friends regularly – if I didn't I'd feel super lonely just being 'mum'. The main reason why I can have a level of my old life is because I fully trust my husband to look after our baby boy. It is hard but I 'let go' of the controlling side that's in me and I take a back seat so I can have my free time. I run through things my husband needs to know and let him get on with things in his own way. Everyone needs a break from being a 'mummy'. Make sure you have your time too – you will be a better mummy for it!

Lucy – Mum of Finley (1)

✸ ✸ ✸

I have recently taken up running twice a week. I also do reflexology once a month and have my brows done monthly.

Vix – Mum of Harry (2)

✳ ✳ ✳

I run or go for an early walk three to four times a week with my dog. The freedom of it being me and him and the time to decompress and mentally go through my tick lists really helps set me up for the day.

Beth – Mum of Rosie (3)

✳ ✳ ✳

Getting my nails and lashes done monthly is a non-negotiable for me. It allows me to feel pampered and to have some peace away from home and work.

Sophie – Mum of Alfie (1)

✳ ✳ ✳

Always remember that you are a couple and make time for each other. Take advantage of doting grandparents and loved ones to go on dates and cheeky nights away. This makes your relationship stronger and happier parents.

Dawn – Mum of Sam (35) and Adam (31)

✳ ✳ ✳

As a stay-at-home mum, my 'me time' is spent tidying and sorting the house or I make it to the supermarket to do the food shopping. I get my hair cut once every three to four months and treat myself to a garden centre lunch every now and again. My husband often takes our daughter out for a bike ride or to his mum's so I can have some me time also.

Amber – Mum of Mollie (3)

✳ ✳ ✳

Even if it's popping to do the food shop on your own, always make time for you. Leave baby with somebody and run a nice bath and relax. Myself and my partner try and do a date night once a month just to connect with each other again, even if it's cooking a lovely meal together, putting the phones down and chatting.

Jess – Mum of Arlo (3) and Luna (10 months)

✳ ✳ ✳

I love to go for a long soak in the bath with a candle and a book just for half an hour to switch off and unwind.

Becca – Mum of Grayson (8 months)

✳ ✳ ✳

Gym/yoga/hiking; generally anything where I'm alone and releasing endorphins.

Lydia – Mum of Mila (3)

✳ ✳ ✳

Have a bath! I ask my husband to look after our daughter for an hour and run myself a bath with music, face mask and plenty of bubbles.

Meg – Mum of Polly (7 months)

✳ ✳ ✳

I go for a walk and a coffee on my own once a week. I don't mind when, but it has to happen. Just being out of the house and alone gives me the healing power I need.

Abi – Mum of Oliver (5) and 7 months pregnant

HANDLING OVERWHELM

Advice on how to handle feeling overwhelmed:

- Write a to do list or action plan – focus on what you can control. You can't spin all of the plates at once.

- Take a deep breath and step away.

- Remember that this feeling won't last, it is only temporary.

- Talk to loved ones about your worries and what they can do to help; delegation can really help and induce some calm.

- Take some time out and try to switch off – try getting out for a walk, doing your favourite hobby or having a pamper session.

- Take a sensory break – consider your senses and how overwhelmed they can get. Just switching off the radio or the TV can bring the pressure down that you are feeling in that moment.

- Have a code word with your partner for when you need to tap out and walk away.

- Write or record it out. Getting out your worries and fears either on paper or in a recording it can make a huge difference and help you plan and rationalise things in a more manageable way.

- If the mum rage starts bubbling and you are worried about your actions, it is okay to walk out of the room and leave your little one for a moment just to calm down.

Being overwhelmed is natural! Your whole life has changed and you are navigating finding a new normal. It can feel all-consuming and the mum rage can start bubbling; working out your triggers and how to regain your calm will make things easier.

Every mum gets overwhelmed, no matter how well others seem to be coping with life and appear to 'have it all'.

Try not to get stuck in perfectionism. Eject those negative thoughts and focus on you and what is important at that time.

Write it out:

_____
_____
_____
_____
_____
_____
_____
_____
_____
_____
_____
_____
_____
_____
_____
_____
_____
_____
_____

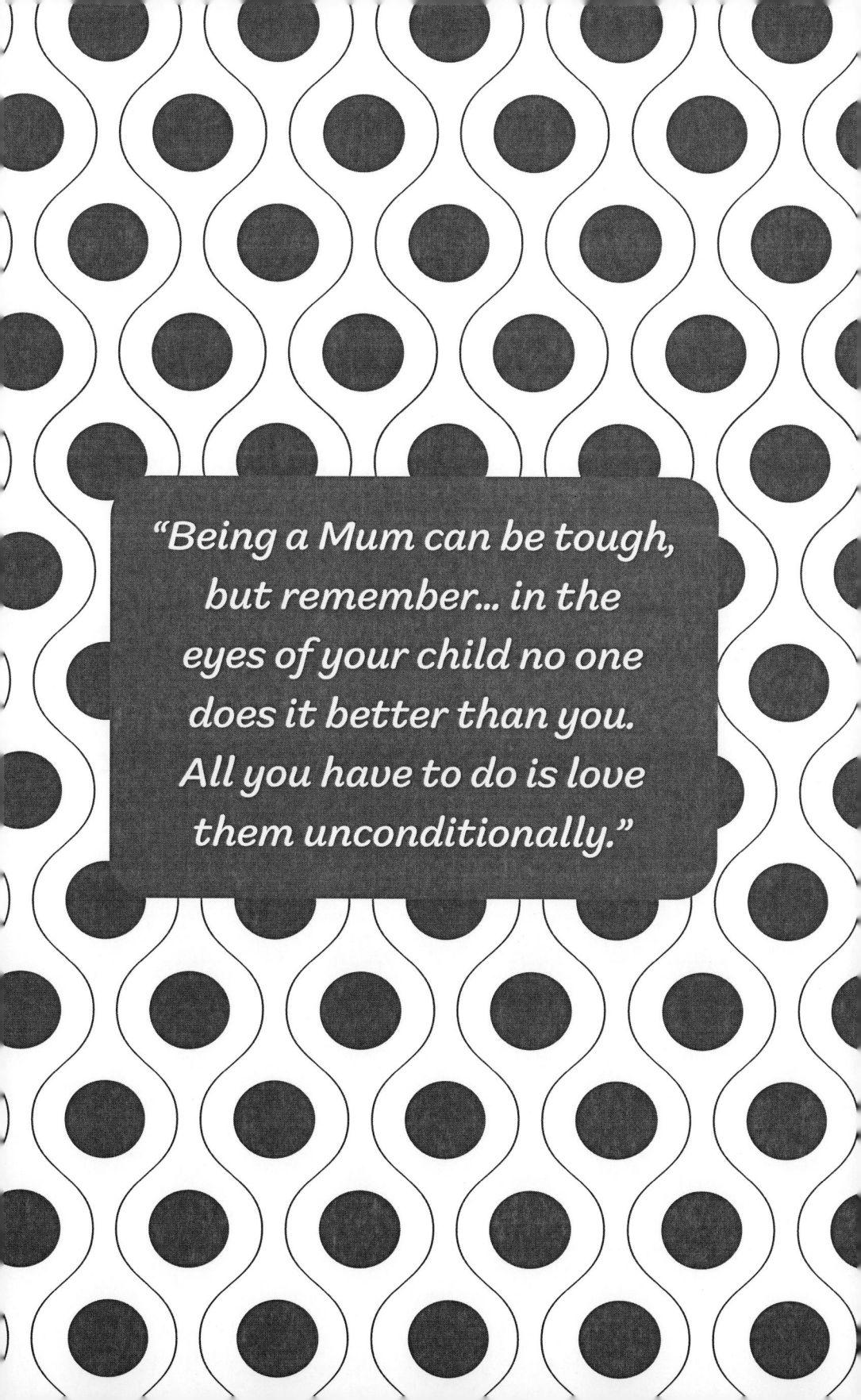

"Being a Mum can be tough, but remember... in the eyes of your child no one does it better than you. All you have to do is love them unconditionally."

Daily Journal

Date: _____

Daily Journal

Date: _____

Daily Journal

Date: _____

Daily Journal

Date: _____

Daily Journal

Date: _____

Daily Journal

Date: _____

Daily Journal

Date: _____

Weekly Check-In

Date: _____

Top 3 things I did this week:

_____

_____

_____

Milestones:

This week I felt:

Next week I would like to:

_____

_____

_____

Things I am proud of this week:

Things to celebrate:

Things to let go of:

My ranking of the week:

☆ ☆ ☆ ☆ ☆

JOURNAL: WEEK FIVE

Daily Journal

Date: _____

Daily Journal

Date: _____

Daily Journal

Date: _____

Daily Journal

Date: _____

Daily Journal

Date: _____

Daily Journal

Date: _____

Daily Journal

Date: _____

JOURNAL: WEEK SIX

Weekly Check-In

Date: _____

Top 3 things I did this week:

_____

_____

_____

This week I felt:

Milestones:

Next week I would like to:

_____

_____

_____

Things I am proud of this week:

Things to celebrate:

Things to let go of:

My ranking of the week:

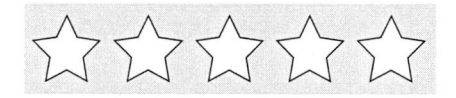

☆ ☆ ☆ ☆ ☆

JOURNAL: WEEK SIX

81

Daily Journal

Date: _____

Daily Journal

Date: _____

Daily Journal

Date: _____

Daily Journal

Date: _____

Daily Journal

Date: _____

Daily Journal

Date: _____

Daily Journal

Date: _____

JOURNAL: WEEK SEVEN

Weekly Check-In

Date: _____

Top 3 things I did this week:

_____

_____

_____

This week I felt:

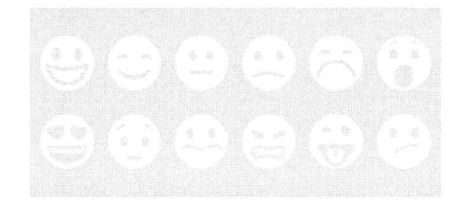

Milestones:

Next week I would like to:

_____

_____

_____

Things I am proud of this week:

Things to celebrate:

Things to let go of:

My ranking of the week:

JOURNAL: WEEK SEVEN

Daily Journal

Date: _____

Daily Journal

Date: _____

_____
_____
_____
_____
_____
_____
_____
_____
_____
_____
_____
_____
_____
_____
_____
_____
_____
_____
_____
_____
_____
_____
_____
_____
_____

Daily Journal

Date: _____

Daily Journal

Date: _____

Daily Journal

Date: _____

Daily Journal

Date: _____

Daily Journal

Date: _____

Weekly Check-In

Date: _____

Top 3 things I did this week:

_____

_____

_____

Milestones:

This week I felt:

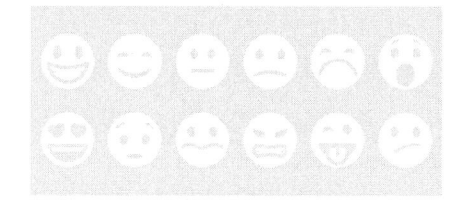

Next week I would like to:

_____

_____

_____

Things I am proud of this week:

Things to celebrate:

Things to let go of:

My ranking of the week:

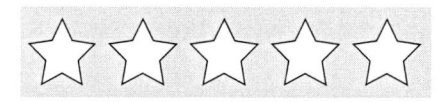

☆ ☆ ☆ ☆ ☆

JOURNAL: WEEK EIGHT

MUM HACKS

- Pull baby's vest down, not up... this avoids poop in their hair.
- Clipping baby's vest over one shoulder can stop vests dunking in their nappies.
- A portable white noise machine is really useful when out and about.
- Try a baby wrap or sling in the house as well as out and about.
- Cut fingernails when baby is sleeping or being fed.
- Help baby understand day and night, keep things loud and bright in the day and dark and quieter at night.
- Make sure YOU stay hydrated; breastfeeding especially can make you very dehydrated. Keep snacks handy too!
- In the early days, remember babies are often only hungry, wet, tired or windy. Go through this checklist and it could help work out what they need.
- If you have fruit going off, it's best to try freezing it or stewing it. It can be great as a yoghurt topper or on porridge. It also works well as a pudding with a crumbled oat bar on top.
- Try setting boundaries for visiting loved ones; make it work for you, not them.
- Invest in a slow cooker. Once baby is down, you will have a hot meal that involves limited prep.
- If baby is very distressed or frustrated, try getting outside or stick them in the bath – the change of scenery does wonders.
- Seal bath toys with glue to stop water going stale inside them.
- Give baby your T-shirt or sleep with their cot sheet for a night or two to help with separation anxiety.
- If you or your baby are feeling really overwhelmed, try deep breathing whilst you hold them. It can really help calm you both.
- Try a toy strap for high chairs for when you are out and about.
- If you have a fussy eater, try adding a little apple puree or grated apple to things like spaghetti Bolognese.

- Fold the top of the nappy down to protect the umbilical cord from being rubbed and help it to dry out.
- Keep your wounds dry and clean. Always reach out to your healthcare professional for help if you have any worries.
- Keep up with your pelvic floor exercises.
- White noise for bedtime: it can mimic being in the womb.
- Have changing items like wipes and nappies in a few different rooms in your home.
- If baby doesn't like bath-time, try distracting them with things like bubbles or putting a towel over them to keep them warm.
- Don't panic about formula – if you switch brands, baby will be okay.
- Cutting up a swim noodle and placing it at the top of doors stops them being slammed and fingers getting caught.
- Try tummy time little and often.
- Raising baby's crib or mattress at one end so it is at an angle can help with reflux or when they have a cold.
- Give your baby naked time, its great for their skin.
- If you can, try to avoid blue light with your little one at least an hour before bed; it can over-stimulate them and make them trickier to settle at bedtime.
- Try warming the Moses basket with a hot water bottle to make the transfer easier – just don't leave it in there!
- Only get a small selection of toys out at a time and then after nap time change them for a new set. This will help keep your child's interest and insure they aren't overwhelmed by too much choice.
- If your little one is tantrumming, screaming, your children are squabbling, you may get those anxious overwhelming feelings come bubbling up. Pause, take a breath and remember that big reactions cause big reactions – try to be the calm in their chaos.
- An oat bath can be brilliant for calming itchy skin from chicken pox or eczema. Try adding half a cup of oats to a clean sock, tie it around the tap and run the bath water through it. Beware of any allergies!
- Lay a towel on the changing mat to help keep baby warm and clean up any accidents.

- Double-up bedding with a waterproof mattress protector between layers to make night-time accidents easier to clean up.
- Buy several of your baby's comforters. They are easily lost and it makes washing them easier if there is always a spare.
- Building your children's toys before you give them on birthdays and Christmas can not only limit stress but it lets your little one play with it straight away.
- Keep toys like puzzles in zip lock bags: easy storage with easy access, and you are less likely to lose pieces.
- Have a portable place mat in your changing bag for weaning little ones; it's great for hygienic finger eating and it stops plates from sliding around.
- Try using glow sticks in the bath or giant pompoms for easy entertainment.
- Stained whites? Try leaving them in the sun, it can naturally bleach items.
- Blended cereals can make great sand… And it's edible, so no need to worry if your little one samples it.
- If your baby won't take medication through a syringe, try putting it in a bottle top/teat.
- Try a no thank you bowl when weaning, it can stop a lot of mess.
- Toothpaste can help get permanent marker off wooden furniture.
- If you have a picky eater, try making them a smoothie.
- A swim noodle can stop your little one from falling out of bed if tucked under the sheet.

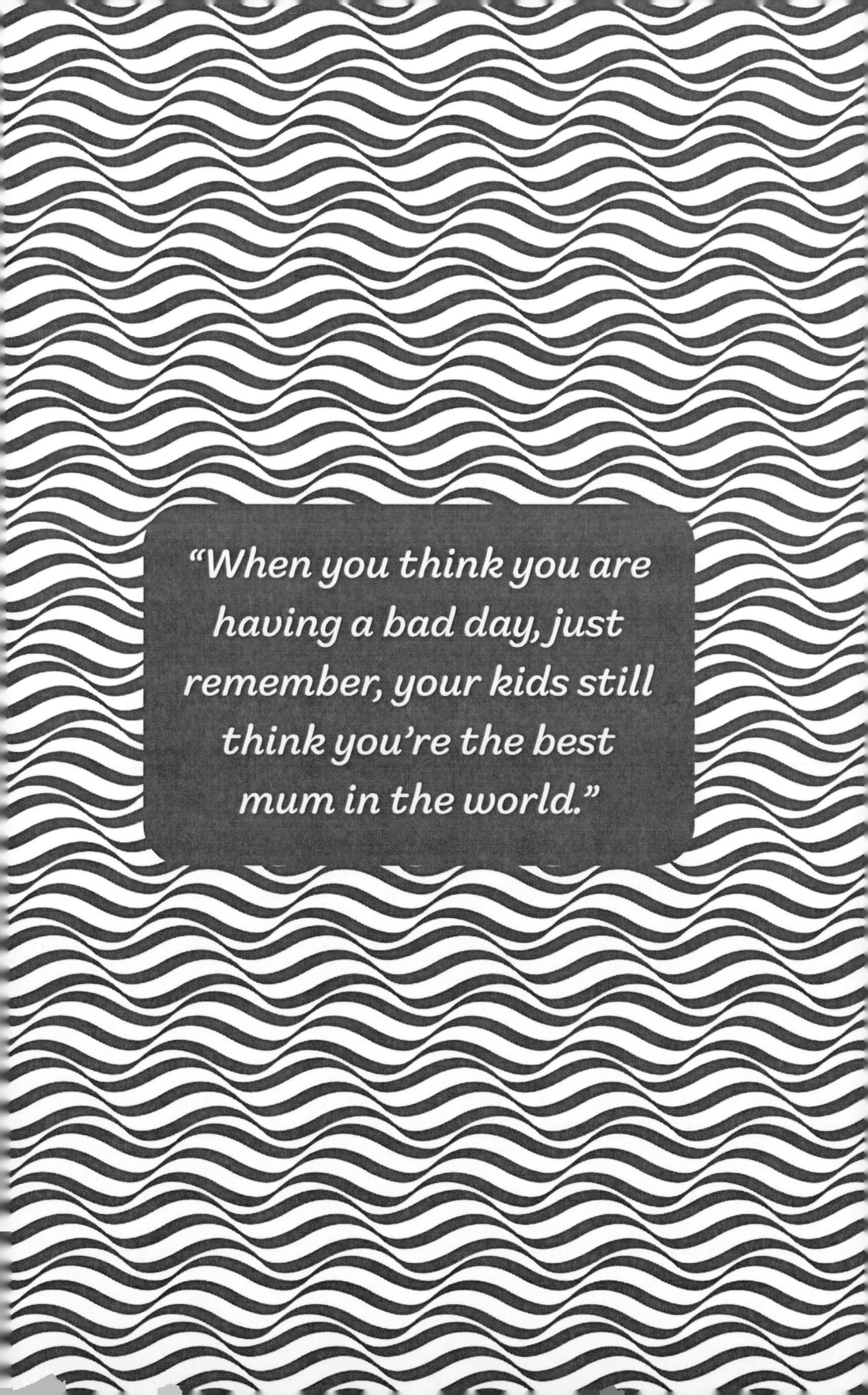

"When you think you are having a bad day, just remember, your kids still think you're the best mum in the world."

Daily Journal

Date: _____

Daily Journal

Date: _____

Daily Journal

Date: _____

Daily Journal

Date: _____

Daily Journal

Date: _____

Daily Journal

Date: _____

Daily Journal

Date: _____

Weekly Check-In

Date: _____

Top 3 things I did this week:

_____

_____

_____

Milestones:

This week I felt:

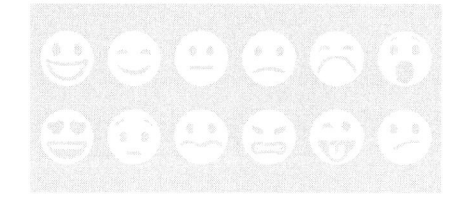

Next week I would like to:

_____

_____

_____

Things I am proud of this week:

Things to celebrate:

Things to let go of:

My ranking of the week:

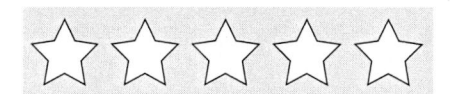

☆ ☆ ☆ ☆ ☆

JOURNAL: WEEK NINE

Daily Journal

Date: _____

Daily Journal

Date: _____

Daily Journal

Date: _____

JOURNAL: WEEK TEN

Daily Journal

Date: _____

Daily Journal

Date: _____

Daily Journal

Date: _____

_____
_____
_____
_____
_____
_____
_____
_____
_____
_____
_____
_____
_____
_____
_____
_____
_____
_____
_____
_____
_____
_____
_____
_____
_____

Daily Journal

Date: _____

Weekly Check-In

Date: _____

Top 3 things I did this week:

_____

_____

_____

Milestones:

This week I felt:

Next week I would like to:

_____

_____

Things I am proud of this week:

Things to celebrate:

Things to let go of:

My ranking of the week:

☆ ☆ ☆ ☆ ☆

JOURNAL: WEEK TEN

Daily Journal

Date: _____

Daily Journal

Date: _____

Daily Journal

Date: _____

Daily Journal

Date: _____

Daily Journal

Date: _____

JOURNAL: WEEK ELEVEN

Daily Journal

Date: _____

Daily Journal

Date: _____

Weekly Check-In

Date: _____

Top 3 things I did this week:

_____
_____
_____

This week I felt:

Milestones:

Next week I would like to:

_____
_____
_____

Things I am proud of this week:

Things to celebrate:

Things to let go of:

My ranking of the week:

☆ ☆ ☆ ☆ ☆

JOURNAL: WEEK ELEVEN 125

Daily Journal

Date: _____

Daily Journal

Date: _____

Daily Journal

Date: _____

Daily Journal

Date: _____

Daily Journal

Date: _____

Daily Journal

Date: _____

Daily Journal

Date: _____

Weekly Check-In

Date: _____

Top 3 things I did this week:

_____

_____

_____

This week I felt:

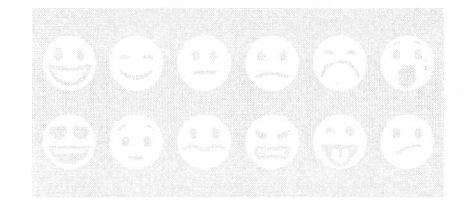

Milestones:

Next week I would like to:

_____

_____

_____

Things I am proud of this week:

Things to celebrate:

Things to let go of:

My ranking of the week:

JOURNAL: WEEK TWELVE

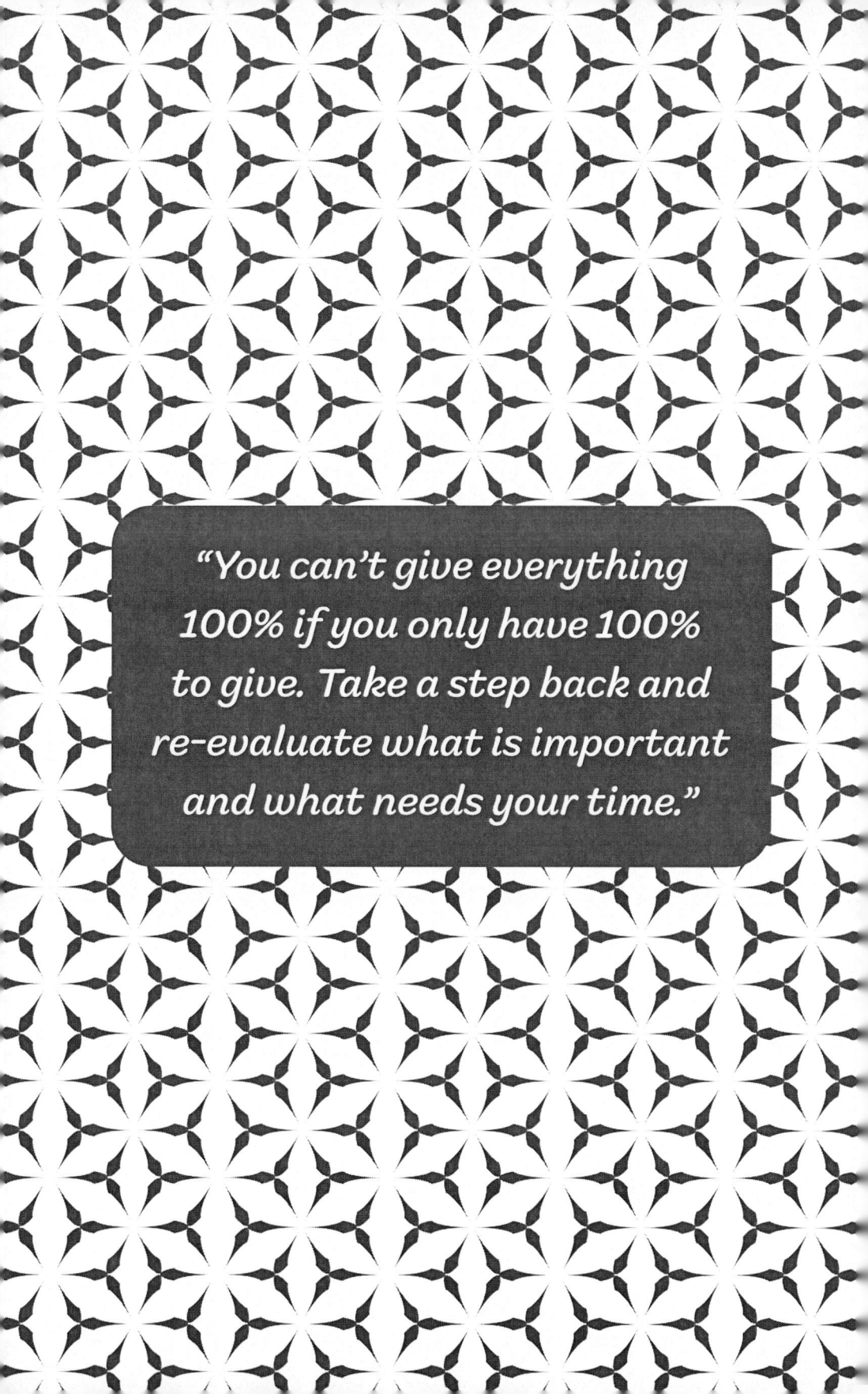

"You can't give everything 100% if you only have 100% to give. Take a step back and re-evaluate what is important and what needs your time."

SIGNS OF POSTNATAL DEPRESSION/ANXIETY AND HOW TO SEEK HELP

- A constant feeling of sadness or feeling very low in yourself.
- Lack of enjoyment and no interest in doing things you would usually enjoy.
- Lack of energy, feeling exhausted and tired all of the time.
- Unable to sleep at night and feeling sleepy and tired during the day.
- Difficulty bonding with your baby or lack of interest in your baby.
- Withdrawing from contact with other people.
- Fear of leaving the house.
- Having panic attacks.
- Fast breathing and irregular heartbeat.
- Nausea, sweating or hot flushes.
- Headaches, back aches or other types of ache.
- Problems concentrating and making decisions.
- Frightening thoughts – for example, about hurting your baby.

A lot of women do not realise they have postnatal depression or postnatal anxiety. It can develop over time, sometimes even after you go back to work or after baby turns 1 or older.

Try to give yourself permission to feel your feelings: they are valid. Asking for help isn't a sign of weakness or failure, it is a sign of strength, love and determination to fight for you and your family.

Call your Doctors Immediately if:

- You have frightening thoughts about hurting your baby or yourself – these can be scary and daunting, but people with these sorts of thoughts rarely harm and hurt their baby.
- You are thinking about **suicide** and **self-harm**.
- You develop unusual thoughts and delusions or have hallucinations (this could be seeing and hearing things that are not real, like hearing voices).

You aren't alone. Don't hide and struggle, thinking that the problem will go away and you will get better. These feelings can often continue for months or years; they can get worse if nothing is done. Depression is treatable. There are so many ways to treat it, and you can and will get better with the right help.

Partners and fathers can also often become depressed after the arrival of a baby. It is important that they also seek help and don't struggle alone.

'REAL LIFE MUMS' WHO KNEW THEY NEEDED HELP WHEN...

I knew I was struggling when I confided in a friend who was also a first-time mum and I spoke to her for advice and help. I used to cry a lot and get so frustrated over the littlest of things. I had to have an emergency C-section and Grayson was rushed to NICU for the first 24 hours. I think the trauma from all of that hit me after a couple of weeks of being home! Having loved ones to confide in really helped me.

Becca – Mum of Grayson (8 months)

✳ ✳ ✳

I realised I was physically frozen on the sofa with the baby on the other side of the room in his Moses basket. Cameron had been sleeping, I had been watching TV. But once he started to stir, I was unable to lift my head to look at him. I didn't want to look him in they eye or chat and poison him with my negative thoughts. I didn't want to look and find I had yet another parenting task to complete. I didn't want to have to pick him up; I was too tired. I didn't want to raise my heart rate by getting off the sofa and find myself in another panic attack. I wanted the sofa the swallow me up and for him to disappear. That's when I knew I needed someone experienced to gently show me how to exist just being around my baby. Once I was gently nudged into holding him, cooing and simply enjoying his company, everything started to fall into place.

Sarah – Mum of Cameron (2)

✳ ✳ ✳

I wouldn't say it was a massive thing, to the point of needing help, but after my second child was born, the second new-born phase hit me with blues more than the first (I don't think I had it the first time). I believe this was due to the sudden separation from my first, nothing to do with little Emi. Jess was no longer my tiny baby! She was so grown up and independent and did amazingly whilst I was away (first time I've been away and something I massively dreaded) – I couldn't be prouder, but oh my goodness, it hit me like a slap in the face. Just lasted a day or two but speaking it out loud really helped and I just let the tears flow – you literally can't control them, they needed to come out.

Vikki – Mum of Jessica (2) and Emilia (2 months)

✳ ✳ ✳

I knew needed help when I would hysterically cry when it was time to feed because the pain made my toes curl in agony!

Sam – Mum of Arlo (2)

✳ ✳ ✳

My husband was about to go for his first night away for a gig with a friend which was a Covid-delayed event – Eleanor was only a month old, I think. I got out of the shower and was stood in my bedroom when I looked down to see both nipples dripping milk, blood dripping down my thigh, and then my hormones hit me with a rush of crying as I knew I would be on my own that night. I felt out of control of my body and I wasn't 'Emma' anymore. I didn't know who I was but I hated what was going on. Worse still, my husband saw me in this state – I felt so embarrassed, which is crazy when I think back now. Like I said, I felt like I lost control of my own body. I had the most precious baby which my incredible body had made so I knew I had to get a grip and get my shit together! My husband, seeing me at this low point, was also an absolute rock to reassure me and get me through this stage!

Emma – Mum of Eleanor (2)

✳ ✳ ✳

I didn't have baby blues, although I had a five-week-old when we went into lockdown, which was daunting. I did miss not being able to have the support/go-to groups, but I found a Facebook group with mums of babies born in the same month, so they really helped. I guess now as a stay-at-home mum I feel like I have the baby blues; sometimes the only people I speak to are Mollie's nursery teacher and Mollie! I suffered massively from separation anxiety when we came out of lockdown and it took a lot of courage for me to let Mollie even go to grandparents' houses to stay over. We took the decision to put her in nursery so we could both have time apart and she could meet other children and I could meet other adults. Even though Mollie is at nursery four days a week, I don't feel like I have a social life; sadly, only on my phone with people. I have lots of mum friends, but we rarely meet due to money and children. There are times when I feel lonely; I feel like I can't talk about it, though, as I am lucky to be in a position not to have to work.

Amber – Mum of Mollie (3)

✳ ✳ ✳

I dealt with motherhood initially really well. Even when baby girl wouldn't latch, we just moved onto to another way of feeding, no troubles either way. Around two months into motherhood, I had a full blown identity crisis and cut myself a proper mum cut. It didn't help! (Don't cut your hair on the fly.) To be honest, I'm still trying to figure myself out now, three years on – but what's the rush?

Lydia – Mum of Mila (3)

✳ ✳ ✳

I was fortunate enough not to suffer from postnatal depression. However, I did have massive issues with catastrophising. I don't think the fact I had a baby in lockdown helped, but I also know my worries were unhealthy. I went through a phase where I couldn't be away from my baby or leave her with anyone except my husband as I was convinced someone was going to snatch her. My mum took her for a walk round the block and was gone five minutes, and it was absolute hell. I was told I needed time to myself but I was so worried about something happening to my beautiful baby that I never let anyone help me. When she started nursery I put on her forms that they weren't allowed to take her off site for walks as again I envisioned people snatching her if they weren't looking. One day I drove past to a meeting and saw all the little babies on a big red baby pram bus going for a walk. My instant thought was how they all looked so cute and happy, but then this was quickly followed by sadness that my little girl was missing out through my own fears. That day I signed the form to say she was allowed out, and although it was hard and scared me it was the day I realised I had to put my own fears and worries aside, otherwise she would never experience fun and happy adventures she deserved to in life. I still struggle sometimes now but I deal with it by rationalising and doing everything I can to keep my girls safe but whilst still letting them be children and having fun.

Margo – Mum of Matilda 3 and Delilah (6 months)

✽ ✽ ✽

I remember getting home from the hospital with my first baby after a pretty traumatic birth, put him down in his car seat in the lounge and thought, 'What on earth do I do now?' We were in Covid lockdown, I had nobody else in the house other than my fiancé. It was so hard. I had to force myself to go out for strolls just to leave the house. I struggled with breastfeeding as it just hurt so much but I kept putting pressure on myself to do it. It was hard, and I felt so guilty because this was all I ever wanted, so why wasn't I happy? With the support of my partner and family, we got through. Baby number 2 came along two years later and I felt like I was back to square one, but this time I knew that it was okay to give her a bottle as she didn't take to the boob; it was okay if I had days where I felt sad and wanted to sit and eat chocolate; and most importantly it was okay to ask for help. Once we all found our own routine it just started to click. I was starting to talk openly about how I was feeling, and things got easier. There is always light at the end of the tunnel! I struggle now with trying to accept my new body which has changed so much, but actually... it created the two most amazing humans. Us woman are incredible; we just don't always give ourselves the credit we deserve.

Jess – Mum of Arlo (3) and Luna (10 months)

✽ ✽ ✽

Breastfeeding was very difficult due to my son's tongue tie. There wasn't enough staff (no feeding specialists) on the ward the night I gave birth to guide me on how to feed my son, or to check over his latch. I was simply told to try formula. I didn't mind swapping to formula, but I struggled with this emotionally, especially when my milk came in after a few days.

Courtney – Mum of Rafi (4 months)

✽ ✽ ✽

No one really talks about when pregnancies don't go to plan. I went into labour at 24 weeks. My baby boy was born and it was a long and scary three-month stay in hospital, including a heart operation at four weeks old. I don't think I suffered from the baby blues as I don't think I had time between hospital visits, expressing and trying to keep the house under a vague form of control. I found the lead-up to his first birthday hard. But after his birthday, I was fine. Like a weight had been lifted of my shoulders. When Mason came home it felt like he just slotted into our lives. But the bond took a very long time to properly form. Everyone used to say you know your baby's cry but I didn't for a very long time. You go into automatic mode, making bottles, feeding, changing, sleeping, seeing people. The bond does eventually come and it's so worth it. Just keep doing what you're doing and don't be afraid to ask for help.

Chloe – Mum of Mason (1)

✽ ✽ ✽

After a dreamy first two weeks with my new-born son, it felt like everything came crashing down. I suddenly started to avoid my son, not wanting to touch him or feed him. I would leave him with his dad and procrastinate by cleaning until I had to breastfeed him. I felt this intense worry and anxiousness, I couldn't eat and I couldn't see a way out of it. It felt like there was no end in sight from this dark tunnel I felt I was in. Small things would tip me over the edge, I would catastrophize everything and pinned a lot of my parenting happiness on how well he slept and whether or not I breastfed.

I was teary throughout these days and felt every emotion under the sun in just one day. My head didn't feel like my own. Luckily, my husband spotted it was something more than baby blue and arranged help. The health visitor was brilliant, as was my doctor. I needed that help and I'm so thankful I opened up.

Rachel – Mum of Leo (2)

"Being a parent is like folding a fitted sheet: no one really knows how to do it."

Daily Journal

Date: _____

Daily Journal

Date: _____

Daily Journal

Date: _____

Daily Journal

Date: _____

Daily Journal

Date: _____

Daily Journal

Date: _____

Daily Journal

Date: _____

Weekly Check-In

Date: _____

Top 3 things I did this week:

_____
_____
_____

This week I felt:

Milestones:

Next week I would like to:

_____
_____
_____

Things I am proud of this week:

Things to celebrate:

Things to let go of:

My ranking of the week:

☆ ☆ ☆ ☆ ☆

JOURNAL: WEEK THIRTEEN

Daily Journal

Date: _____

Daily Journal

Date: _____

Daily Journal

Date: _____

Daily Journal

Date: _____

Daily Journal

Date: _____

Daily Journal

Date: _____

Daily Journal

Date: _____

Weekly Check-In

Date: _____

Top 3 things I did this week:

_____

_____

_____

Milestones:

This week I felt:

Next week I would like to:

_____

_____

_____

Things I am proud of this week:

Things to celebrate:

Things to let go of:

My ranking of the week:

☆ ☆ ☆ ☆ ☆

JOURNAL: WEEK FOURTEEN

Daily Journal

Date: _____

Daily Journal

Date: _____

Daily Journal

Date: _____

Daily Journal

Date: _____

Daily Journal

Date: _____

Daily Journal

Date: _____

Daily Journal

Date: _____

JOURNAL: WEEK FIFTEEN

Weekly Check-In

Date: _____

Top 3 things I did this week:

_____
_____
_____

Milestones:

This week I felt:

Next week I would like to:

_____
_____
_____

Things I am proud of this week:

Things to celebrate:

Things to let go of:

My ranking of the week:

☆ ☆ ☆ ☆ ☆

JOURNAL: WEEK FIFTEEN

Daily Journal

Date: _____

Daily Journal

Date: _____

Daily Journal

Date: _____

Daily Journal

Date: _____

_____
_____
_____
_____
_____
_____
_____
_____
_____
_____
_____
_____
_____
_____
_____
_____
_____
_____
_____
_____
_____
_____
_____

Daily Journal

Date: _____

Daily Journal

Date: _____

Daily Journal

Date: _____

Weekly Check-In

Date: _____

Top 3 things I did this week:

_____
_____
_____

This week I felt:

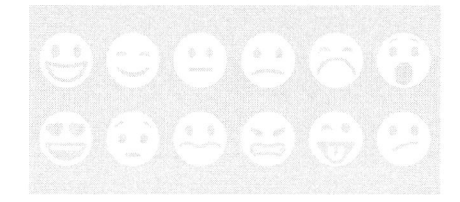

Milestones:

Next week I would like to:

_____
_____
_____

Things I am proud of this week:

Things to celebrate:

Things to let go of:

My ranking of the week:

☆ ☆ ☆ ☆ ☆

JOURNAL: WEEK SIXTEEN 175

Daily Journal

Date: _____

Daily Journal

Date: _____

Daily Journal

Date: _____

JOURNAL: WEEK SEVENTEEN

Daily Journal

Date: _____

Daily Journal

Date: _____

Daily Journal

Date: _____

Daily Journal   Date: _____

JOURNAL: WEEK SEVENTEEN

Weekly Check-In

Date: _____

Top 3 things I did this week:

_____

_____

_____

This week I felt:

Milestones:

Next week I would like to:

_____

_____

Things I am proud of this week:

Things to celebrate:

Things to let go of:

My ranking of the week:

JOURNAL: WEEK SEVENTEEN

Daily Journal

Date: _____

Daily Journal

Date: _____

Daily Journal

Date: _____

Daily Journal

Date: _____

Daily Journal

Date: _____

Daily Journal

Date: _____

Daily Journal

Date: _____

Weekly Check-In

Date: _____

Top 3 things I did this week:

_____
_____
_____

This week I felt:

Milestones:

Next week I would like to:

_____
_____
_____

Things I am proud of this week:

Things to celebrate:

Things to let go of:

My ranking of the week:

☆ ☆ ☆ ☆ ☆

JOURNAL: WEEK EIGHTEEN

Daily Journal

Date: _____

_____
_____
_____
_____
_____
_____
_____
_____
_____
_____
_____
_____
_____
_____
_____
_____
_____
_____
_____
_____
_____
_____
_____
_____
_____
_____

Daily Journal

Date: _____

Daily Journal

Date: _____

Daily Journal

Date: _____

Daily Journal

Date: _____

Daily Journal

Date: _____

Daily Journal

Date: _____

Weekly Check-In

Date: _____

Top 3 things I did this week:

_____

_____

_____

This week I felt:

Milestones:

Next week I would like to:

_____

_____

_____

Things I am proud of this week:

Things to celebrate:

Things to let go of:

My ranking of the week:

JOURNAL: WEEK NINETEEN

Daily Journal

Date: _____

Daily Journal

Date: _____

Daily Journal

Date: _____

Daily Journal

Date: _____

Daily Journal

Date: _____

Daily Journal

Date: _____

Daily Journal

Date: _____

Weekly Check-In

Date: _____

Top 3 things I did this week:

_____

_____

_____

This week I felt:

Milestones:

Next week I would like to:

_____

_____

_____

Things I am proud of this week:

Things to celebrate:

Things to let go of:

My ranking of the week:

☆ ☆ ☆ ☆ ☆

JOURNAL: WEEK TWENTY

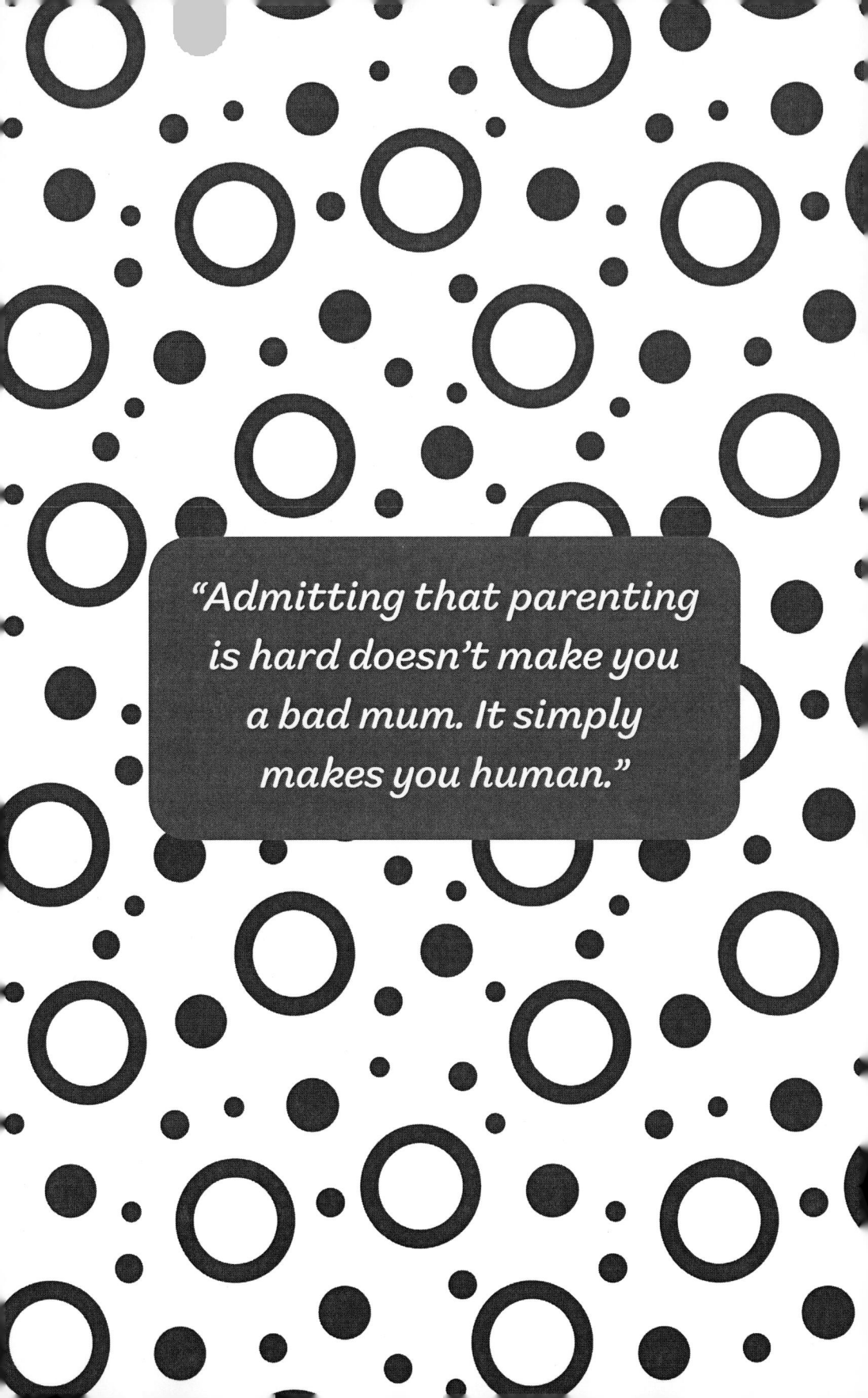

"Admitting that parenting is hard doesn't make you a bad mum. It simply makes you human."

MANAGING MUM BURNOUT

Burnout is very common for all mums, no matter the age of your child or children. You are juggling housework, life admin, friends, family, your relationship, work and more. Here are a few handy tips on how to handle burnout and how to make managing the mental load a little easier.

- Ask for help, be honest with your partner, friends and loved ones. Delegate things that can ease the pressure on you. It may not be done to your standard but the help is there – so utilise it!
- Set boundaries: it is okay to say no to things you don't want to do.
- Put yourself and your family's needs before others.
- Create a routine: this will help with forward planning.
- Schedule in 'you time' to allow you to decompress – try to make this non-negotiable.
- Lower your expectations and standards – housework can wait, the world won't end if you don't clean the cooker today.
- Try to remember that if it isn't a problem for you it shouldn't be a problem for others.
- Take a social media detox. It can be harmful to consistently compare yourself to others; no one's life is perfect and no one has the perfect child who never cries and sleeps like an angel.
- Try to improve your sleep schedule: just an extra half an hour can make a world of difference.
- Get organised: try decluttering that cupboard that is overflowing or tidy your wardrobe.
- Let go of the guilt: it's okay to have a beige meal here and there, it's okay to relax during nap time and it's okay to leave the life admin an extra day or two or till next week.

How can you help limit your burnout:

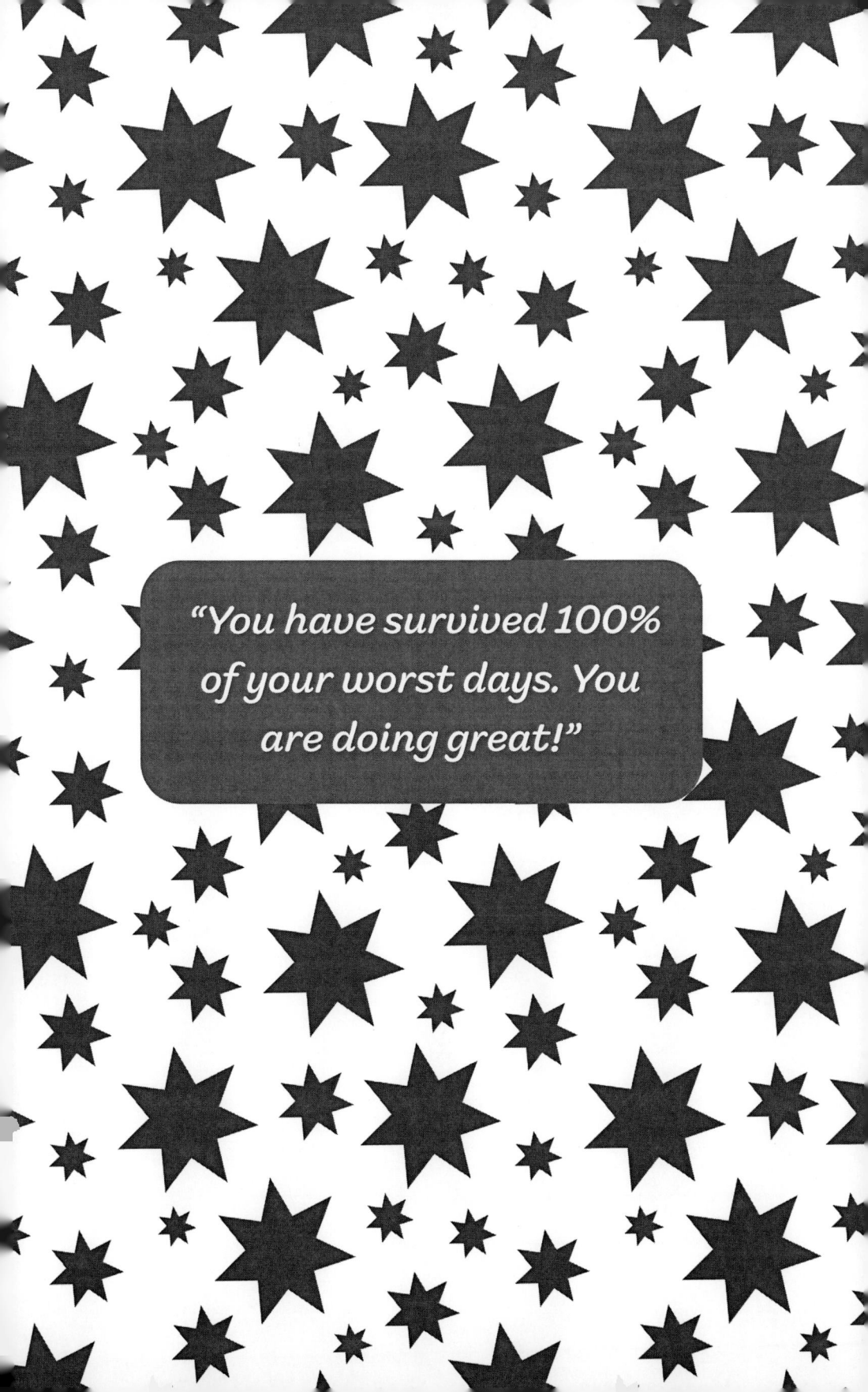

"You have survived 100% of your worst days. You are doing great!"

Daily Journal

Date: _____

Daily Journal

Date: _____

Daily Journal

Date: _____

Daily Journal

Date: _____

Daily Journal

Date: _____

JOURNAL: WEEK TWENTY-ONE

Daily Journal

Date: _____

Daily Journal

Date: _____

Weekly Check-In

Date: _____

Top 3 things I did this week:

_____

_____

_____

This week I felt:

Milestones:

Next week I would like to:

_____

_____

_____

Things I am proud of this week:

Things to celebrate:

Things to let go of:

My ranking of the week:

☆ ☆ ☆ ☆ ☆

JOURNAL: WEEK TWENTY-ONE

Daily Journal

Date: _____

Daily Journal

Date: _____

Daily Journal

Date: _____

Daily Journal

Date: _____

Daily Journal

Date: _____

Daily Journal

Date: _____

Daily Journal

Date: _____

Weekly Check-In

Date: _____

Top 3 things I did this week:

_____

_____

_____

This week I felt:

Next week I would like to:

_____

_____

_____

Milestones:

Things I am proud of this week:

Things to celebrate:

Things to let go of:

My ranking of the week:

☆ ☆ ☆ ☆ ☆

JOURNAL: WEEK TWENTY-TWO   227

Daily Journal

Date: _____

Daily Journal

Date: _____

Daily Journal

Date: _____

Daily Journal

Date: _____

Daily Journal

Date: _____

JOURNAL: WEEK TWENTY-THREE

Daily Journal

Date: _____

Daily Journal

Date: _____

JOURNAL: WEEK TWENTY-THREE

Weekly Check-In

Date: _____

Top 3 things I did this week:

_____

_____

_____

This week I felt:

Milestones:

Next week I would like to:

_____

_____

_____

Things I am proud of this week:

Things to celebrate:

Things to let go of:

My ranking of the week:

☆ ☆ ☆ ☆ ☆

JOURNAL: WEEK TWENTY-THREE

Daily Journal

Date: _____

Daily Journal

Date: _____

Daily Journal

Date: _____

JOURNAL: WEEK TWENTY-FOUR

Daily Journal

Date: _____

Daily Journal

Date: _____

Daily Journal

Date: _____

Daily Journal

Date: _____

Weekly Check-In

Date: _____

Top 3 things I did this week:

_____
_____
_____

This week I felt:

Milestones:

Next week I would like to:

_____
_____
_____

Things I am proud of this week:

Things to celebrate:

Things to let go of:

My ranking of the week:

JOURNAL: WEEK TWENTY-FOUR

Has anyone asked you recently if you were bottle-fed or breast-fed as a baby?

Has anyone asked if you were born vaginally or via C-section?

Has anyone asked if your mum had an epidural?

Has anyone asked you what age you were potty-trained or if you co-slept with your mum or if you were rocked to sleep when you were a baby?

All of these worries may seem so huge at the moment, but in the long run it doesn't matter.

Be kind to yourself.

Trust your gut and do your best.

Motherhood is a journey.

EXPECTATIONS VS REALITY

Waiting for your baby to arrive can feel like an eternity: you sit and wonder what they will be like, you plan and imagine your new life and the adventures and memories you will have with them. It is a mixture of wonderful and terrifying, and more often than not you have these huge expectations as to what it will be like – and the reality is nothing like it. That can be quite a big adjustment to get your head around, and unburdening your mind can often help you adjust to your new normal.

Advice on what to write:
- How was labour different to what you expected?
- How has your life changed since the arrival of baby?
- How is parenting different to what you expected?
- What are you enjoying that you didn't expect to?
- What are you not enjoying that you didn't expect to not enjoy?
- What do you want to change and go back to doing now baby is here?
- How has your relationship changed?
- How are you different as a person?
- What is harder than you expected?

Expectations:

Reality:

EXPECTATIONS VS REALITY

> "Bad moments don't make bad mums."

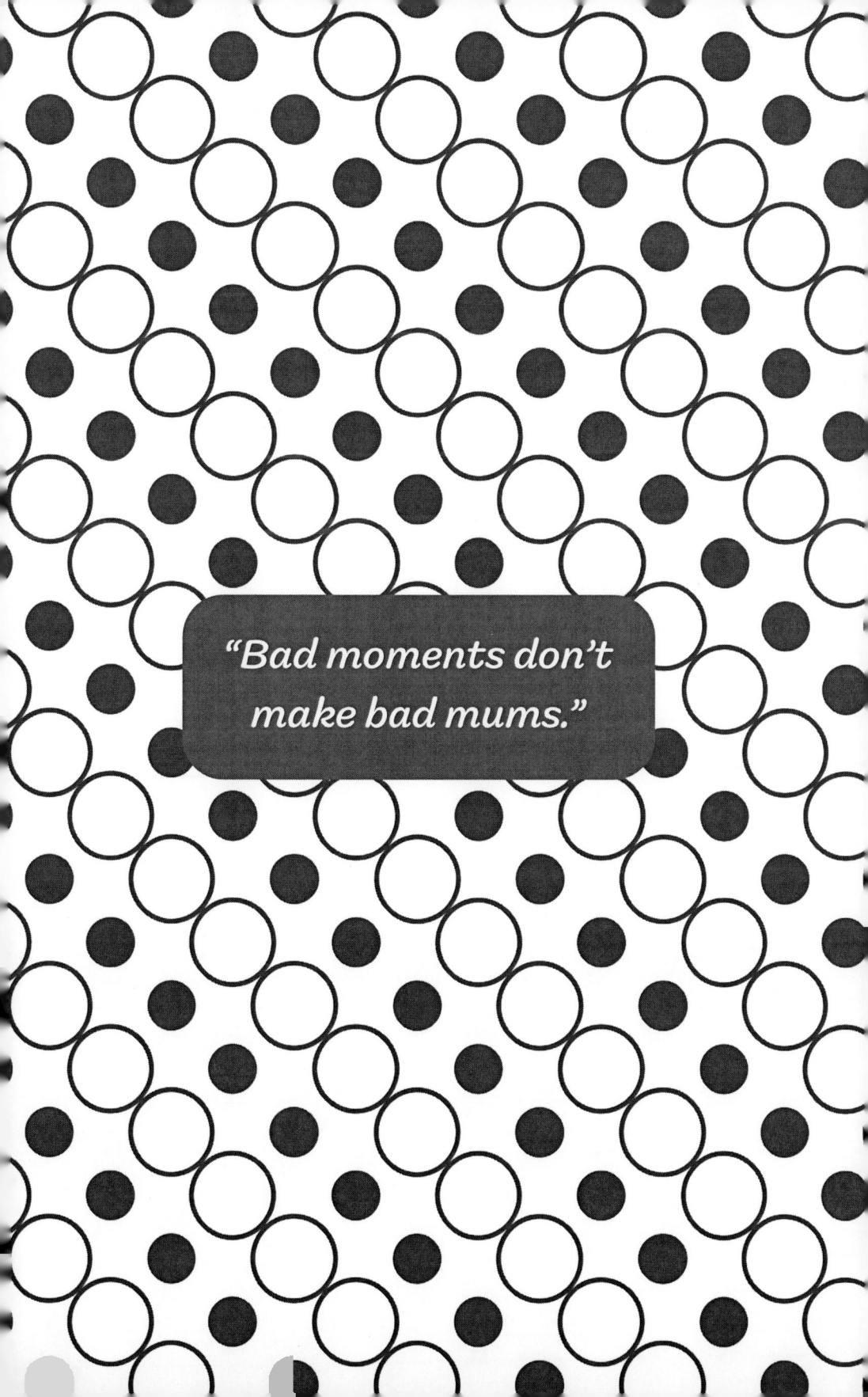

Daily Journal

Date: _____

Daily Journal

Date: _____

Daily Journal

Date: _____

Daily Journal

Date: _____

Daily Journal

Date: _____

Daily Journal

Date: _____

Daily Journal

Date: _____

Weekly Check-In

Date: _____

Top 3 things I did this week:

_____

_____

_____

Milestones:

This week I felt:

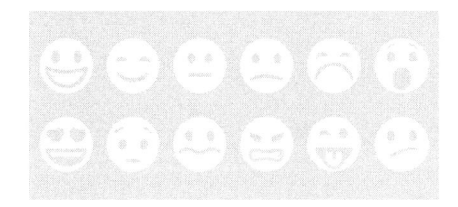

Next week I would like to:

_____

_____

_____

Things I am proud of this week:

Things to celebrate:

Things to let go of:

My ranking of the week:

☆ ☆ ☆ ☆ ☆

JOURNAL: WEEK TWENTY-FIVE

Daily Journal

Date: _____

Daily Journal

Date: _____

Daily Journal

Date: _____

Daily Journal

Date: _____

Daily Journal

Date: _____

Daily Journal

Date: _____

Daily Journal

Date: _____

Weekly Check-In

Date: _____

Top 3 things I did this week:

_____

_____

_____

This week I felt:

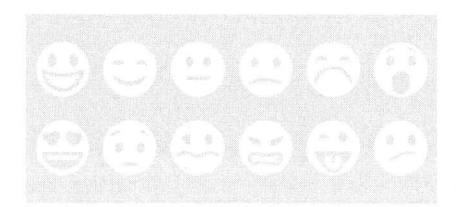

Milestones:

Next week I would like to:

_____

_____

_____

Things I am proud of this week:

Things to celebrate:

Things to let go of:

My ranking of the week:

☆ ☆ ☆ ☆ ☆

JOURNAL: WEEK TWENTY-SIX

Daily Journal

Date: _____

Daily Journal

Date: _____

Daily Journal

Date: _____

Daily Journal

Date: _____

Daily Journal

Date: _____

Daily Journal

Date: _____

Daily Journal

Date: _____

Weekly Check-In

Date: _____

Top 3 things I did this week:

_____

_____

_____

This week I felt:

Milestones:

Next week I would like to:

_____

_____

Things I am proud of this week:

Things to celebrate:

Things to let go of:

My ranking of the week:

JOURNAL: WEEK TWENTY-SEVEN

Daily Journal

Date: _____

JOURNAL: WEEK TWENTY-EIGHT

Daily Journal

Date: _____

Daily Journal

Date: _____

Daily Journal

Date: _____

Daily Journal   Date: _____

_____
_____
_____
_____
_____
_____
_____
_____
_____
_____
_____
_____
_____
_____
_____
_____
_____
_____
_____
_____
_____
_____
_____
_____
_____
_____
_____
_____
_____
_____

Daily Journal

Date: _____

_____
_____
_____
_____
_____
_____
_____
_____
_____
_____
_____
_____
_____
_____
_____
_____
_____
_____
_____
_____
_____
_____
_____
_____
_____

Daily Journal

Date: _____

Weekly Check-In

Date: _____

Top 3 things I did this week:

_____
_____
_____

Milestones:

This week I felt:

Next week I would like to:

_____
_____
_____

Things I am proud of this week:

Things to celebrate:

Things to let go of:

My ranking of the week:

☆ ☆ ☆ ☆ ☆

JOURNAL: WEEK TWENTY-EIGHT

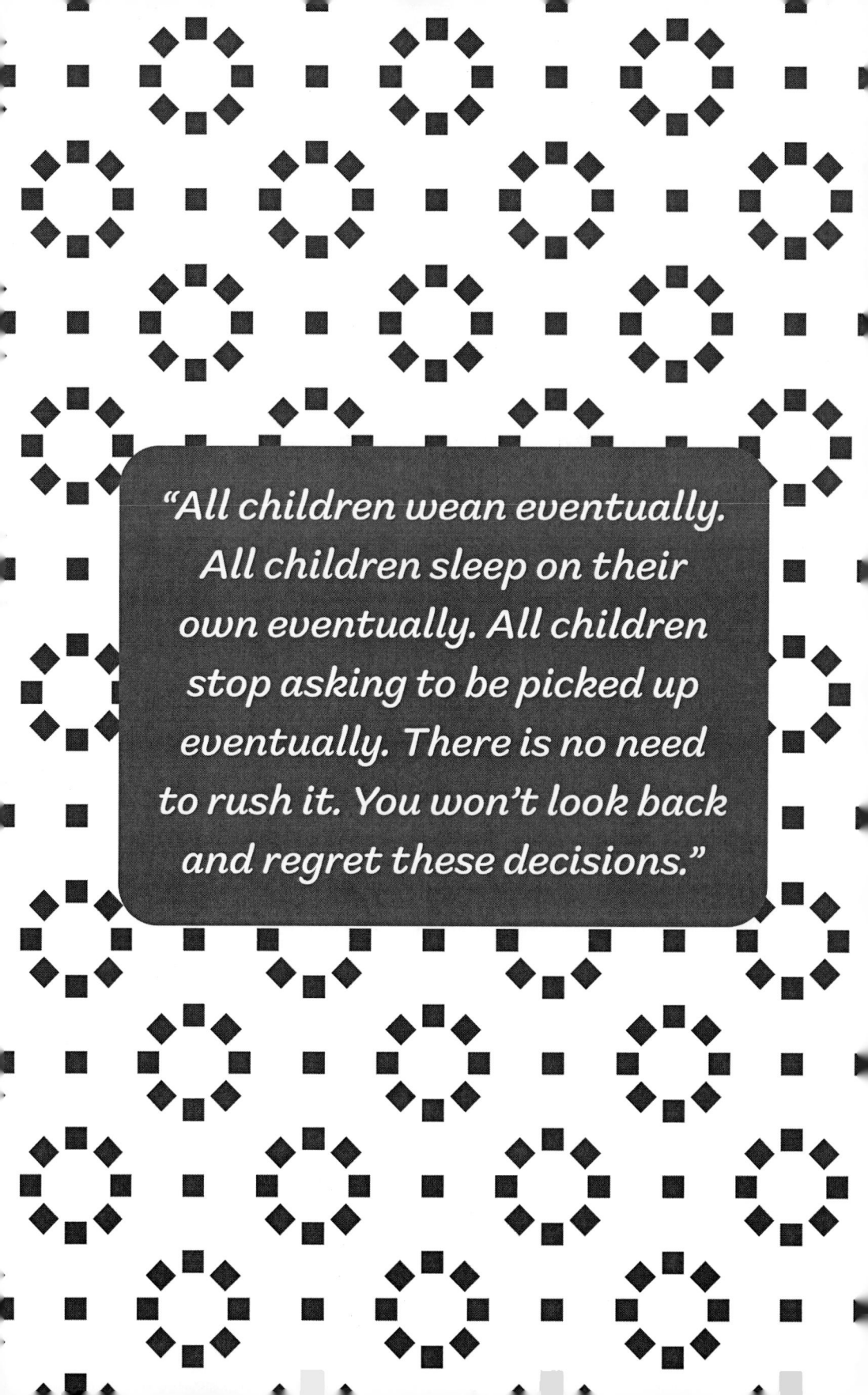

"All children wean eventually. All children sleep on their own eventually. All children stop asking to be picked up eventually. There is no need to rush it. You won't look back and regret these decisions."

AFFIRMATIONS

Affirmations can be a fantastic way to breathe positivity back into your life and to overcome self-sabotaging thoughts whilst building your confidence and self-love. If you can, try to say your chosen affirmations daily. You could also encourage your children to eventually start using affirmations: they can be a very powerful tool for anyone, of any age.

•

I am a good mother

•

I know how to take care of my baby and what is best for them and me

•

I am a powerful, loving and calm being

•

I am a dedicated and loving mother

•

My connection with my baby grows stronger every day

•

I am surrounded by those who love, support and respect me

•

I am good enough in all that I do

I am worthy of receiving love

My body is strong, beautiful and has done incredible things

I am learning to be a mother every day

I have the strength to take care of all my baby's needs

I love myself no matter what

The way I choose to parent is the best choice for my family

I can face difficult situations with courage and conviction

I am enough

Everything is a phase, and it will get easier

I allow myself to be me and give myself time to take care of myself

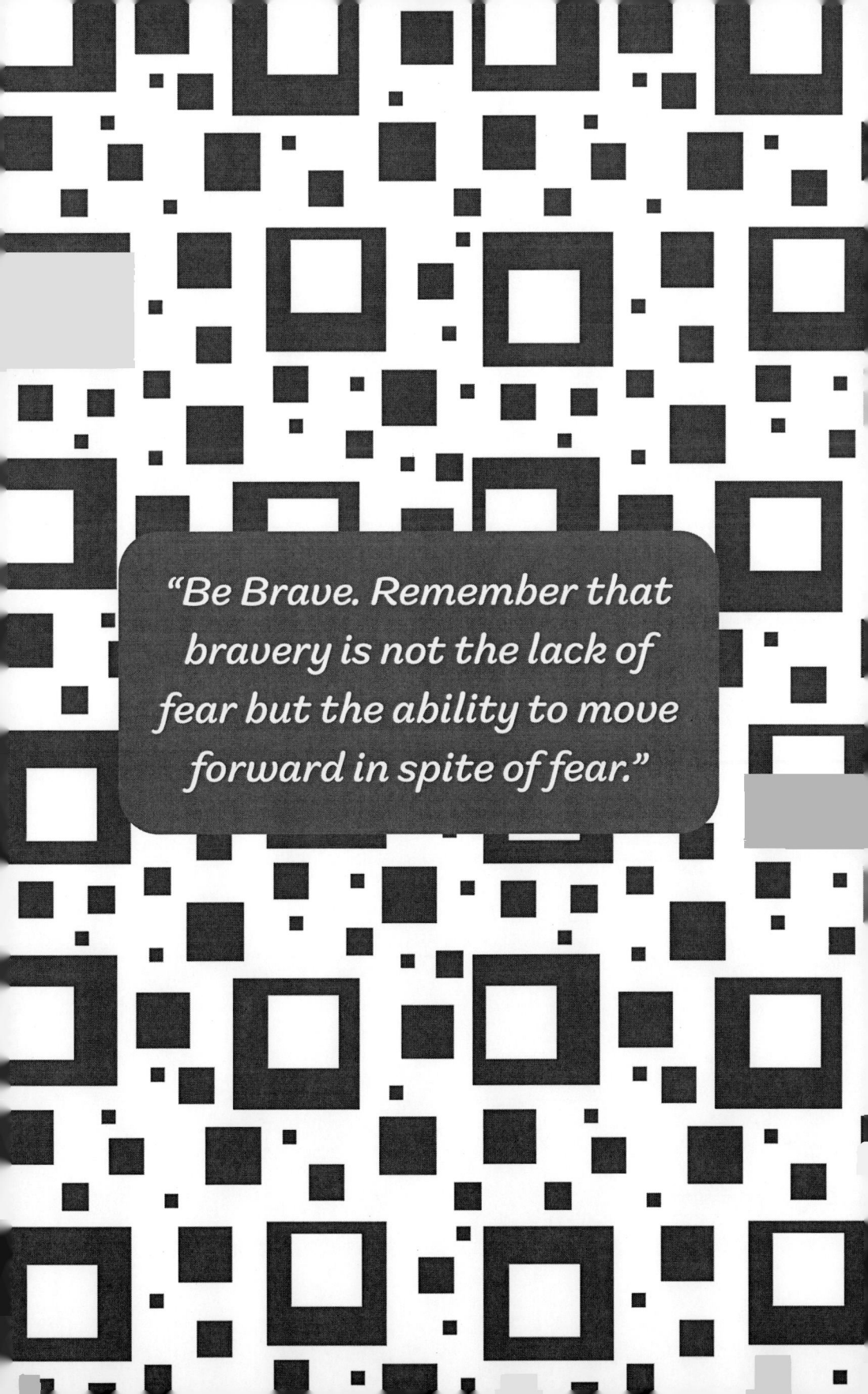

"Be Brave. Remember that bravery is not the lack of fear but the ability to move forward in spite of fear."

Daily Journal

Date: _____

Daily Journal

Date: _____

Daily Journal　　　　　Date: _____

Daily Journal

Date: _____

Daily Journal

Date: _____

Daily Journal

Date: _____

Daily Journal

Date: _____

Weekly Check-In

Date: _____

Top 3 things I did this week:

_____

_____

_____

This week I felt:

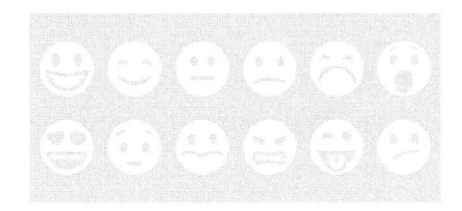

Milestones:

Next week I would like to:

_____

_____

_____

Things I am proud of this week:

Things to celebrate:

Things to let go of:

My ranking of the week:

☆ ☆ ☆ ☆ ☆

JOURNAL: WEEK TWENTY-NINE

Daily Journal

Date: _____

Daily Journal

Date: _____

Daily Journal

Date: _____

Daily Journal

Date: _____

Daily Journal

Date: _____

Daily Journal

Date: _____

Daily Journal

Date: _____

Weekly Check-In

Date: _____

Top 3 things I did this week:

_____

_____

_____

Milestones:

This week I felt:

Next week I would like to:

_____

_____

Things I am proud of this week:

Things to celebrate:

Things to let go of:

My ranking of the week:

Daily Journal

Date: _____

Daily Journal

Date: _____

Daily Journal

Date: _____

Daily Journal

Date: _____

Daily Journal

Date: _____

Daily Journal

Date: _____

Daily Journal

Date: _____

Weekly Check-In

Date: _____

Top 3 things I did this week:

_____

_____

_____

Milestones:

This week I felt:

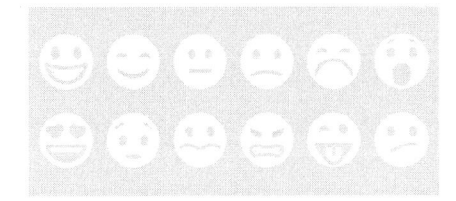

Next week I would like to:

_____

_____

_____

Things I am proud of this week:

Things to celebrate:

Things to let go of:

My ranking of the week:

Daily Journal

Date: _____

Daily Journal

Date: _____

Daily Journal

Date: _____

Daily Journal

Date: _____

Daily Journal

Date: _____

_____
_____
_____
_____
_____
_____
_____
_____
_____
_____
_____
_____
_____
_____
_____
_____
_____
_____
_____
_____
_____
_____
_____
_____
_____
_____
_____
_____

Daily Journal

Date: _____

Daily Journal

Date: _____

Weekly Check-In

Date: _____

Top 3 things I did this week:

_____

_____

_____

Milestones:

This week I felt:

Next week I would like to:

_____

_____

_____

Things I am proud of this week:

Things to celebrate:

Things to let go of:

My ranking of the week:

JOURNAL: WEEK THIRTY-TWO

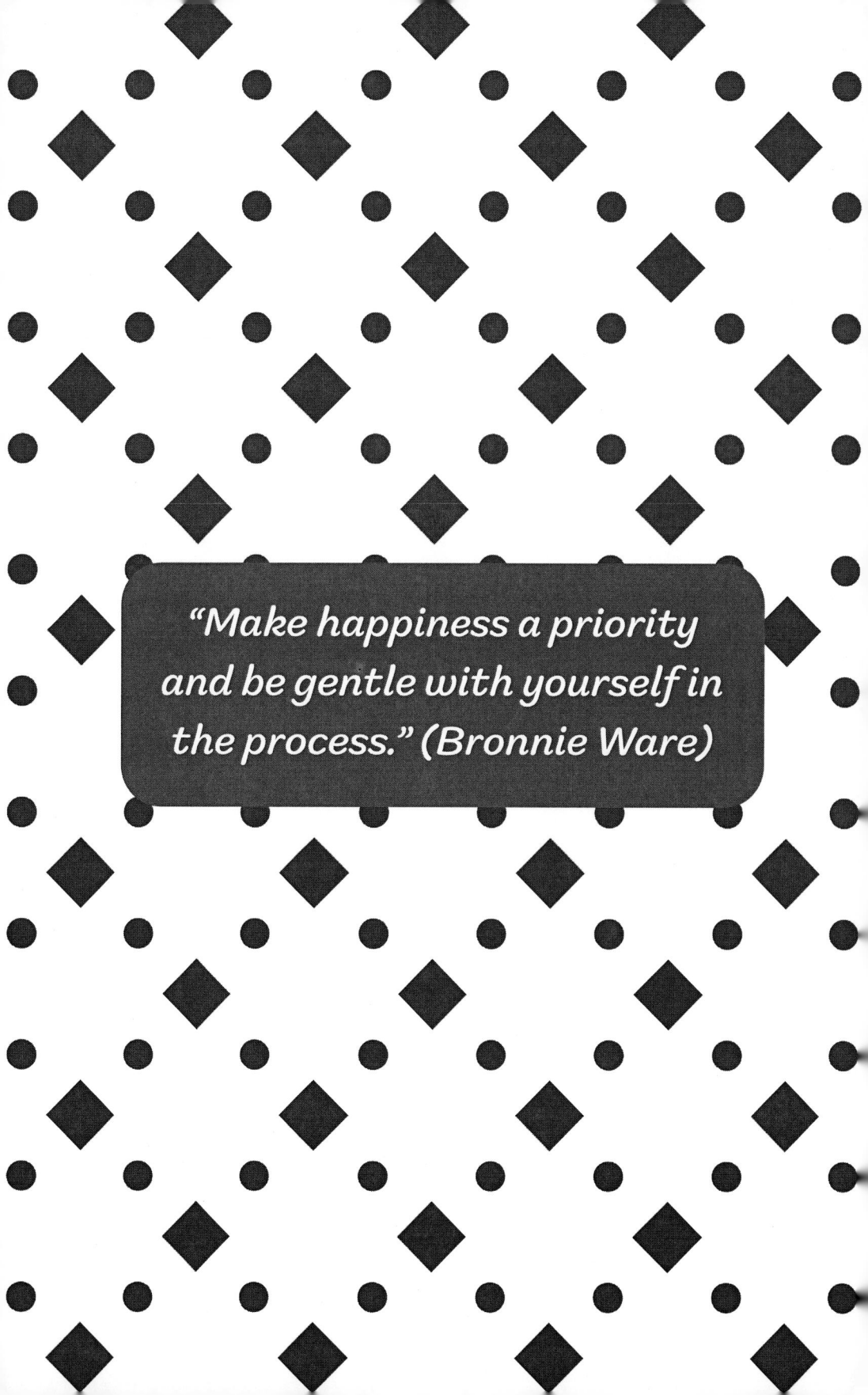

"Make happiness a priority and be gentle with yourself in the process." (Bronnie Ware)

ADVICE FROM 'REAL LIFE MUMS'

It gets easier; you find your rhythm and what works for you as a family. Until then, know that you're not alone and that everything is just a moment in time. Also... no one is judging you. Being a new mum is like being a part of the world's best club. Everyone is there to support you. Open up to those new mums you meet, because they're probably, almost definitely, feeling what you are feeling.

Rachel – Mum of Leo (2)

✳ ✳ ✳

You are doing a great job: try to stop putting pressure on yourself and how your baby is fed. Remember, fed is best and a happy mum= a happy baby.

Sandy – Mum of Annie (31), Nick (34) and Milly (28)

✳ ✳ ✳

Don't put too much pressure on yourself. You will know what's right in your gut. Take any help you can get for dinners, washing, cleaning, etc.

Sam – Mum of Arlo (2)

✳ ✳ ✳

'Comparison is the theft of joy...' Ignore all that nonsense and pressure you see on social media. Do you really think the mum with the perfectly cooked, nutritious, five-veggie patties in her perfect kitchen doesn't have toys, snot and nappies all over her living room floor? Do you really think that mum posting the perfect photo of her little one on the beach isn't in a world of pain dealing with a kid that wants to eat sand and tantrums every two minutes? Do you really think the mum posting a cute photo of her having 'the best cuddles with my poorly angel' hasn't been awake all night, eaten/drank or peed in the past five hours, or

constantly cleaned up vomit and done three washing loads today? Unfollow those pages that made you feel inadequate or forced you into a state of comparison.

Sarah – Mum of Cameron (2)

✢ ✢ ✢

Soak up every second with your baby and don't feel like you have to do everything according to society. Trust your 'mum head' and do what works for you and your baby.

Becca – Mum of Grayson (8 months)

✢ ✢ ✢

Everybody has an opinion (but remember it's just that – an opinion) and everything can feel so worrying that you may feel like you're not enjoying it or living in the moment. I remember the first year of my daughter's life I felt I spent 80% of it worrying about illnesses, sickness bugs, chest infections, etc., and that it was miserable. But putting together an album of her first year made me realise how many incredible memories we had and it reminded me to live in the moment and embrace everything. Children will always get ill just before you go away, they will throw tantrums right at the point you desperately want them to behave, and they will chuck that dinner you spent hours making from scratch on the floor and refuse to eat it – but my best advice is, don't sweat the small stuff or let it consume you, because when you look back it's all the little smiles and moments of love and happiness that you remember.

Margo – Mum of Matilda (3) and Delilah (6 months)

✢ ✢ ✢

So I think what I really struggled with when becoming a mum was losing control of my body and not really knowing what to expect. I had always been a size 8 before falling pregnant, probably due to years of dancing from the age of three and good with healthy eating, but suddenly after birth, I had this weight all over my body, which I thought wouldn't hang around – but it did! I had too many people tell me, 'You will snap back,' but that didn't happen. So I felt very low about my body, as I had very high expectations. My advice: 'Relax and let it go, you have to remind yourself that your body just grew a baby so it's good to let it have a slow recovery'. I was so uptight after my birth! Not being in control of my body was really difficult, with bleeding and milky boobs. I had been given advice like, 'You need huge thick pads after birth because you will bleed loads for months after,' or, 'You need breast pads to soak up all that milk which can spray out of your boobs'. I just didn't feel prepared, and this scared me! I didn't know how heavy the blood would be, how long will it last, blood clots or how will milk be spraying out. My advice: trust your body. Everyone is different; don't overthink it, your body will recover in its own time.

Emma – Mum of Eleanor (2)

✳ ✳ ✳

Don't be afraid to ignore the endless pieces of advice you will receive – some of it is unsolicited, some of it will be wanted. You will be given so much advice, but not everything will work for you and your baby, or be relevant to your situation. It can be so overwhelming at such a vulnerable time.

Courtney – Mum of Rafi (4 months)

✳ ✳ ✳

No one knows your baby better than you! Don't get too hung up on the baby books highlighting what your baby should be doing week by week. You and your baby will find your groove in your own time and at your own pace. Sleep, eating and pooping are unique to each individual baby, and no book can account for all, so trust your instinct and create your own week by week suited for you and your baby.

More than ever, parenting is about teamwork. Sharing the load and supporting one another are paramount. There are no awards for trying to do everything yourself.

Scarlett – Mum of Hugo (2)

✳ ✳ ✳

No matter what everyone tells you, there's no right or wrong way. Do what you as their mum think is right. You can only do your best, and your best is always enough.

Vicki – Mum of Freddie (7) and Millie (5)

✳ ✳ ✳

A helpful piece of advice I would give new mums is things that you think matter don't matter. For example, I know it's all part of the nesting process, but I never washed Mason's clothes before he wore them and that was when he was in hospital and was absolutely fine. His room was not ready and at a year old I would say his room is just about the way I imagined it. As much as I would have liked to have everything ready, that choice was taken away and we coped, and what we didn't have when he came home we could get delivered or family members would go and get for us.

Chloe – Mum of Mason (1)

✳ ✳ ✳

Let go of control. I found it really hard to begin with to keep the house clean, do laundry, put dinner on the table, stay in contact with everybody and meet up with everyone who wanted to see the baby. Let it go and take things one day at a time. You and baby come first. Say no to plans and don't feel guilty. They are only newborns for a few weeks, so enjoy it and spend it cuddling your little one – the housework and everybody else can wait!

Meg – Mum of Polly (7 months)

✳ ✳ ✳

Everyone hears how amazing it is becoming a mum. In part it is true. It is the most magical and precious time, full of pure love, that it's incomparable... But... what no one tells you is that it will also be one of the hardest times of your life, both emotionally and physically. I now know why sleep deprivation is used for torture! For the first three years of each of my kids' life I barely slept three hours a night; glue ear, food intolerances, sickness, bugs, you name it – non-stop! Nursery brings it all home. If I had less than two hours of sleep for six days running (which was a lot), I used to go to the toilet and break down and cry. It was hard. For me, when both turned three, it was like a switch... Life turned easy!! (Although it's taking years for my body to learn to sleep again!)

I have four bits of advice...

1. Sex can't be planned! Grab it when you can! My second baby was a planned C-section, so no chance of a 'tear'... but sex was agony for the first nine months .. I didn't understand why, I thought it was thrush... but it wasn't. It was horrible. It was like losing your virginity over and over again... but I pushed through the pain until eventually, nine months later, it was enjoyable again. And it was soooo worth it!

2. Always trust your instincts. Mother's intuition is a real thing.

3. Always follow through with your threats. It's hard, but the long-term reward is priceless. If you don't follow through, your kids will become more undisciplined.

4. Let someone you trust have your baby overnight on a regular basis from an early age. I didn't let anyone have my oldest until near one year old, and she then struggled with separation anxiety. I had my parents look after my youngest from eight weeks. It was hard for me, but it was right for my baby. It became normal for him, and he experienced no anxiety and developed a close relationship with those I trust. My kids are 'Mummy', 'Mummy', 'Mummy'... and would only develop a close relationship with another person if I wasn't there for them to focus on. It also left time for me to be a wife and a friend instead of a mum.

Claire – Mum of Lia (9) and Jacob (6)

Daily Journal

Date: _____

Daily Journal

Date: _____

Daily Journal

Date: _____

Daily Journal

Date: _____

Daily Journal

Date: _____

Daily Journal

Date: _____

Daily Journal

Date: _____

Weekly Check-In

Date: _____

Top 3 things I did this week:

_____

_____

_____

This week I felt:

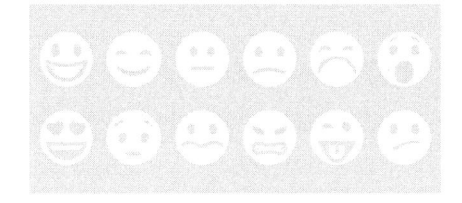

Milestones:

Next week I would like to:

_____

_____

_____

Things I am proud of this week:

Things to celebrate:

Things to let go of:

My ranking of the week:

☆ ☆ ☆ ☆ ☆

JOURNAL: WEEK THIRTY-THREE

Daily Journal

Date: _____

Daily Journal

Date: _____

Daily Journal

Date: _____

JOURNAL: WEEK THIRTY-FOUR

Daily Journal

Date: _____

Daily Journal

Date: _____

Daily Journal

Date: _____

Daily Journal

Date: _____

_____
_____
_____
_____
_____
_____
_____
_____
_____
_____
_____
_____
_____
_____
_____
_____
_____
_____
_____
_____
_____
_____
_____
_____
_____
_____
_____
_____
_____
_____

Weekly Check-In

Date: _____

Top 3 things I did this week:

_____

_____

_____

This week I felt:

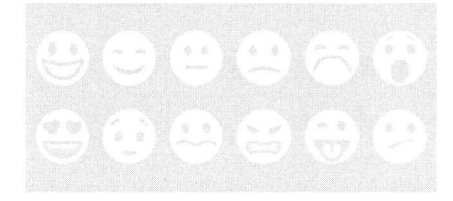

Milestones:

Next week I would like to:

_____

_____

_____

Things I am proud of this week:

Things to celebrate:

Things to let go of:

My ranking of the week:

☆ ☆ ☆ ☆ ☆

Daily Journal

Date: _____

Daily Journal

Date: _____

Daily Journal

Date: _____

JOURNAL: WEEK THIRTY-FIVE

Daily Journal

Date: _____

Daily Journal

Date: _____

Daily Journal

Date: _____

Daily Journal Date: _____

JOURNAL: WEEK THIRTY-FIVE

Weekly Check-In

Date: _____

Top 3 things I did this week:

_____

_____

_____

This week I felt:

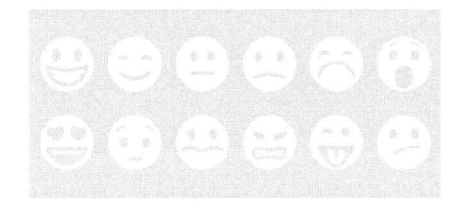

Milestones:

Next week I would like to:

_____

_____

_____

Things I am proud of this week:

Things to celebrate:

Things to let go of:

My ranking of the week:

☆ ☆ ☆ ☆ ☆

JOURNAL: WEEK THIRTY-FIVE

Daily Journal

Date: _____

Daily Journal

Date: _____

Daily Journal

Date: _____

Daily Journal

Date: _____

Daily Journal

Date: _____

Daily Journal

Date: _____

Daily Journal

Date: _____

Weekly Check-In

Date: _____

Top 3 things I did this week:

_____

_____

_____

Milestones:

This week I felt:

Next week I would like to:

_____

_____

_____

Things I am proud of this week:

Things to celebrate:

Things to let go of:

My ranking of the week:

☆ ☆ ☆ ☆ ☆

JOURNAL: WEEK THIRTY-SIX

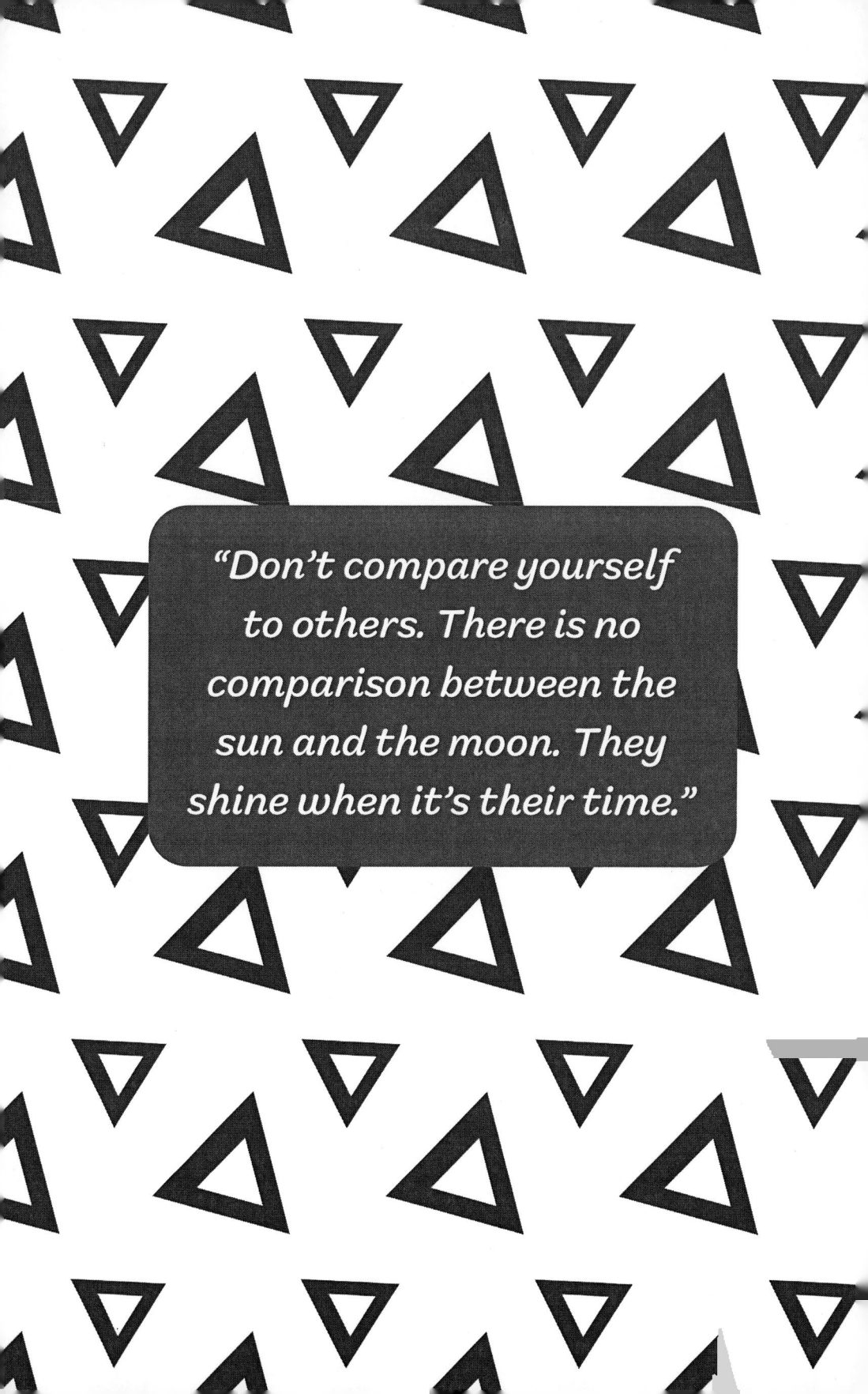

"Don't compare yourself to others. There is no comparison between the sun and the moon. They shine when it's their time."

IDENTITY AND HOW TO FIND YOURSELF AGAIN

No one tells you that when you become a mum you lose part of yourself. Yes, you gain a huge new part to you but you somehow, more often than not, lose a big part of you also. That could be through your career, financial independence, your body, friendships, relationships, dealing with mum judgement, feeding problems, unexpected challenges with your little one and more. You have to navigate this whole new journey, and your needs are always put last. Your identity isn't fixed: it's healthy to change and grow as the years pass. No one is the same person as they were one, two, three or even ten years ago. Find your new groove and own who you want to be and the journey you are on.

There is no right or wrong way to parent; you need to do what works for you and your family. Try to imagine what things would look like if you could do whatever you wanted, how would you feel if you did that gym class or went out for that coffee. Then implement those things step by step and you will gradually gain some of you back. Never forget that all of your feelings are valid and that all mums go through a lot of these feelings at some point.

Here are a few helpful tips on how to reclaim you and your identity:

- Find something for you in every day – sitting down and enjoying a hot coffee, going for a walk or doing your favourite hobby. Try and let your child fit in around you where possible.
- Try looking in the mirror every day and say three nice things to yourself; remember to speak to yourself as you would your best friend.

- Say no to things that don't make you happy. Don't force yourself to go to see people you don't want to or go to things that cause you mental worries and stress.
- If fashion is your dilemma and you don't know how to style your new body or new mum vibe, try finding a few pieces that you love and build from there. Start with a new jacket, a particular pair of shoes or top. Finding a timeless staple that will stay with you for years is always a winner.
- Try to connect with friends – meeting for a walk, going for a drink or dinner, or have a catch up at home over a cuppa or glass of wine.
- Stop comparing yourself to other people and your old self. It's normal not to look the same or not to do the same things as you used to do. Everyone is fighting a battle, whether they share it or not, and everyone is on a different path. Just because one person is out socialising with friends, working and seemingly 'having it all' doesn't mean they are – and it doesn't mean you have to be. Do what makes you happy: stay in, go out – do what works for you!
- Don't force relationships that aren't natural. Just because you both have children doesn't mean you connect as people.
- Give yourself a goal to work to: something to focus on can really help.
- Reconnect with your partner. If you can't go out for a date night, try doing one at home.
- Think about all the positive ways your baby has changed you and what you have accomplished since having them. It's easy to focus on negatives, but in reality you have achieved something utterly remarkable by growing a little human – that needs some celebrating.
- Date yourself – get to know you again. Look back at things you used to love and try doing them again. Look back over the years: did you love art, sport, reading? Is there a language you have always wanted to learn? Get to know you again; and remember, it can take a few attempts to find out what you love!

How can you get your identity back?

Daily Journal

Date: _____

Daily Journal

Date: _____

Daily Journal

Date: _____

Daily Journal

Date: _____

Daily Journal

Date: _____

Daily Journal

Date: _____

Daily Journal

Date: _____

Weekly Check-In

Date: _____

Top 3 things I did this week:

_____

_____

_____

Milestones:

This week I felt:

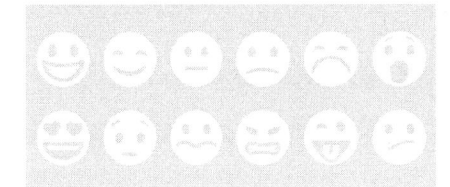

Next week I would like to:

_____

_____

_____

Things I am proud of this week:

Things to celebrate:

Things to let go of:

My ranking of the week:

☆ ☆ ☆ ☆ ☆

JOURNAL: WEEK THIRTY-SEVEN   365

Daily Journal

Date: _____

Daily Journal

Date: _____

Daily Journal

Date: _____

Daily Journal

Date: _____

Daily Journal

Date: _____

Daily Journal

Date: _____

Daily Journal

Date: _____

Weekly Check-In

Date: _____

Top 3 things I did this week:

_____

_____

_____

This week I felt:

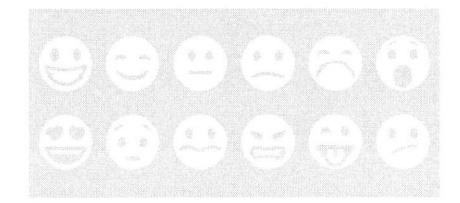

Milestones:

Next week I would like to:

_____

_____

_____

Things I am proud of this week:

Things to celebrate:

Things to let go of:

My ranking of the week:

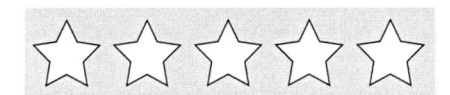

☆ ☆ ☆ ☆ ☆

JOURNAL: WEEK THIRTY-EIGHT

Daily Journal

Date: _____

Daily Journal

Date: _____

Daily Journal

Date: _____

Daily Journal

Date: _____

Daily Journal Date: _____

Daily Journal

Date: _____

Daily Journal

Date: _____

Weekly Check-In

Date: _____

Top 3 things I did this week:

_____

_____

_____

This week I felt:

Milestones:

Next week I would like to:

_____

_____

_____

Things I am proud of this week:

Things to celebrate:

Things to let go of:

My ranking of the week:

JOURNAL: WEEK THIRTY-NINE

381

Daily Journal

Date: _____

Daily Journal

Date: _____

Daily Journal

Date: _____

Daily Journal

Date: _____

Daily Journal

Date: _____

JOURNAL: WEEK FORTY

Daily Journal

Date: _____

Daily Journal

Date: _____

JOURNAL: WEEK FORTY

Weekly Check-In

Date: _____

Top 3 things I did this week:

_____

_____

_____

This week I felt:

Milestones:

Next week I would like to:

_____

_____

_____

Things I am proud of this week:

Things to celebrate:

Things to let go of:

My ranking of the week:

☆ ☆ ☆ ☆ ☆

JOURNAL: WEEK FORTY 389

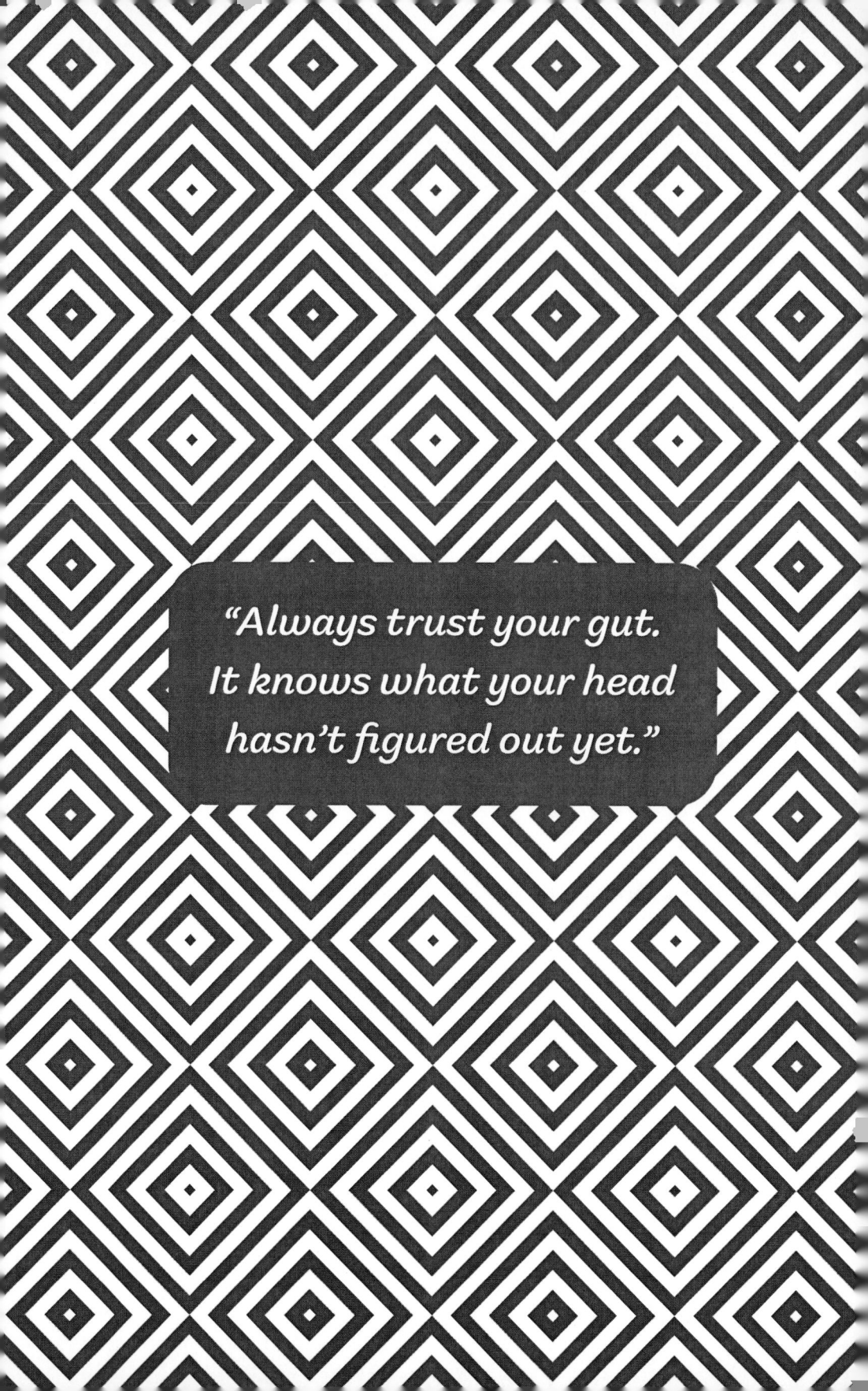

"Always trust your gut. It knows what your head hasn't figured out yet."

BOBBY'S STORY

A 'Real Life Mum's' Journey into Supporting a Child with Additional Challenges

Bobby is my third child. I already had two teenage daughters from a previous relationship before I met Paul, and I wasn't planning on doing it all again. But I did, and so I went from being a teenage mother to a geriatric one (the NHS term, not mine!). I am one of those annoying women who loved pregnancy, and Bobby's was no exception. Despite the odd few weeks of morning sickness, it was a textbook pregnancy. All my check-ups, scans and blood work were all reassuring and there was nothing to worry about. I planned to give birth in the natural baby unit and I often joked about being a 'veteran'.

Like my other two pregnancies, the nine months came and went and I passed my due date. My mother, who we suspected was a bit of a witch, confidently claimed that he would be born on her birthday and be a boy – making him her first grandson.

With the intention to encourage the baby to get a wriggle on, I went into labour after a long country walk. Contractions started in the early evening, and by two in the morning we headed to the hospital. Frustratingly, I wasn't dilated enough, so we were sent back home to ride out the next few hours. Seven in the morning came, and it was time. Clinging to the sides of the car, Paul whisked me to the hospital and this time I stayed.

Much to the annoyance of the midwives, I walked myself to the natural birthing unit as I found this was helping with the contractions. (My top labour advice here is to never let anyone tell you how to position yourself when you are in labour, unless there is a medical emergency. Follow what your body wants, because it's an amazing thing and knows what to do.)

The midwife started to fill up the birthing pool and Paul stood there like a deer in the headlights – all pretty standard, really. Then as I tried to climb into the pool – apologies for the overshare – my waters broke, and they were green. Meconium. My contractions grew fierce and the desire to push was consuming; however, I could no longer stay there. I was quickly chucked into a wheelchair and hurried through the hospital to the main ward. I barely made it to the bed when I went into pushing mode. Bobby was born less than an hour after arriving at the hospital. A boy. On my mum's birthday.

What I remember about the next few hours was how quiet it all was. Bobby didn't cry when he entered the world. It was eerily silent. Due to the meconium, they immediately took him to be checked over. I also remember Paul asking if the baby was okay, and what we had. After what seemed like forever, but was realistically no more than five minutes or so, they put my beautiful son in my arms.

I will never forget that moment. I looked at this tiny face and I instantly noticed these dark pools of brown which had this sense of both wonder and confusion as to what had just happened. I smiled at him and introduced myself as his mummy. During this time, I had two midwives with me, one being a student, and they quickly got to work completing the admin side of things, seeing now how Bobby was fine. The student was being shown how to use the computer and every now and then, they would turn back and ask me a question about my pregnancy or when my contractions started and so forth. Paul went out to call our families.

I want to say that my maternal instincts kicked in straight away and that I noticed something wasn't right – after all, I was this veteran mum, which I kept bragging about – but they didn't. I did notice that his chin seemed on the small side, and that there was a lack of wanting to feed, but I thought I had a chilled baby. The other thing, and with the benefit of hindsight should have been a huge wailing siren going off, was his hypertonia. He couldn't hold his head up — at all! But no one else, apart from my mum, seemed to be concerned. I should trust the professionals, right?

I tried to breastfeed, but it wasn't going well; this was something as a teenage mum I had really struggled with, so I put it down to my inability and not Bobby's. Because of his hypertonia, we were shown how to feed him using the express and syringe feed method — this involves expressing and then using a small plastic syringe to gently feed your baby. The midwives, confident that I had it all under control, allowed us home the next day.

Four days later, I was still struggling to feed him, but he wasn't excessively crying, in fact he had this adorable kitten-like cry which was incredibly endearing. He was so quiet and slept — a lot! Words of wisdom had told me that boys were different to girls, they were more 'relaxed' and they were 'easier'. We persevered with breastfeeding using the syringe method and I had several midwives share their advice on how to get him to latch to the breast, and another, more seasoned, reassured me that bottle feeding is not giving up. Despite this, we found ourselves back in hospital as Bobby had an infection and lost more than 10% of his birth weight.

Bobby was there for a week, and because he was on the premature babies unit due to lack of space on the main ward, we weren't allowed to stay. I was heartbroken. His tiny hands both had cannulas wrapped in bandages which made them look like boxing gloves. I remember this painful, overwhelming need to be with him. I would sob all the way home and all the way back to him. Even now I remember that feeling, the pull to be with him. It was genuinely traumatic.

During his stay, there was a lot of discussion about his chin — or rather lack of it — this is known as micrognathia and it was suspected that Bobby had this. Fortunately, he recovered from his infection, and we got his birth weight back up so were discharged and booked in for a follow up in the March to see how his chin was doing.

Over the next few months, my mum was constantly nagging at me to get Bobby checked over. I kept reassuring her that everything was fine. Yet, by his seven-week review, he still had no muscle tone, so I asked the GP if this was normal. He said it was okay and that babies develop at different speeds. My mother was fuming, but I didn't see the panic as to me Bobby was this adorable baby with the deep brown eyes who just wanted to cuddle all day. To make her happy, I booked an extra appointment with a health visitor. She checked him over and advised me that he was fine and that boys have a tendency to be 'lazy'. Having only had girls, I somewhat accepted this.

But by this point, I was beginning to notice things. For example, Bobby wouldn't grab his feet; he wasn't interested in rolling over; he still couldn't lift his own head; his tongue would stick out cutely when concentrating on his toys, toys he couldn't really hold or even engage with. I commented to Paul that I was having to teach him things that I remember the girls instinctively doing.

Christmas came and went, and the next doctor we saw was at the check-up appointment in March. Unbeknown to us at the time, she is highly respected in her field. The appointment was meant to be a ten-minute review; we were there for an hour and half. We sat down and she asked how we had all been, to which we replied, 'Fine, but we have some concerns.' She listened and then asked to examine Bobby. She played with him while checking him over and asked questions about his general health. I remember watching her trying to read what she was thinking.

We sat down and she kindly said that she agreed that we were right to raise our concerns. She turned to type up her observations, at which point Bobby started crying for his bottle. She turned and kindly asked if that was how he always sounded when hungry? Smiling, we replied with how cute we found his kitten cry. It was at this point that she said that ultimately there was nothing we have failed to do or that there was anything we could have done differently. She believed there was a genetic reason why Bobby wasn't developing as we would expect. Honestly, this was a relief. At last we had been heard.

The next hour involved all three of us having blood tests and answering questions about our medical history. We got the results within three weeks.

At the follow-up, our consultant gently informed us that Bobby had a rare genetic condition known as cri-du-chat and that she never expected to meet someone with it in her career. It was a sporadic mutation and the key indicator is the kitten-like cry. It was when Bobby had become hungry that he gave her the sign of what to look for. The most powerful thing that come from this meeting, and has become a mantra to us, were her words of support: Bobby will do things his own way and will show us all what he is capable of achieving.

Looking back, the next few days seemed to be a blur. We told family and friends straight away, and as you can imagine my mum was relieved that we finally had an answer. I remember almost hiding away in the bedroom with him, not because I was ashamed or upset, but because I needed time to process his diagnosis, to get ready to begin this new journey. All I wanted to do was to protect him and I needed to build up the energy to do this. It was a couple of days before I googled the condition. I am glad I waited, and if you ever find yourself in this position, please give yourself this grace time.

I discovered that the things which were overlooked should have been seen as red flags. For example: lack of muscle tone; the small chin; not being able to successfully breastfeed, which can be an indicator of something more serious; the different-sounding cry, and even the lack of it; excessive sleeping and being an 'easy' baby. At times I had been made to feel like I was being hypervigilant, even paranoid. However, after his diagnosis, I was listened to. I was now the person who the doctors sought for advice and to understand my son's condition. As anticipated, this was the beginning of an extraordinary journey, with just as many highs as there are lows. Fortunately, the lows have become fewer as Bobby has grown and my brown-eyed boy continues to warm my heart every day with 'showing me all the amazing things that he is capable of'.

I feel privileged to be Bobby's mummy and my advice (which is age-old), is that, regardless of whether this is your first or twentieth child, trust your instincts, even if they contradict others. Furthermore, your experience might have similarities to mine, in that you may not have noticed things straight away. If this is the case, I hope that you don't carry any guilt around with you. It doesn't make us bad parents for missing things. For me, I was somewhat blinded by a mother's love and was focused on the positives. I still am today and I won't ever feel guilty for that.

So, if your child is born with special needs, you will have a different normal. It may take some time to adjust to this, and may be lonely, overwhelming, or even funny and exciting at times, but it is a special experience, and our children are incredibly special.

By Emma – Mum to Bobby (aged five)

SIGNS YOUR CHILD COULD HAVE ADDITIONAL CHALLENGES

More often than not there is nothing for you to worry about. Emotions are running high, you are sleep-deprived and as mums we often over-analyse everything. Whether we like it or not, we are always comparing and thinking about when our baby is doing this or that. However, if you are overly concerned – here are some signs to watch out for and how to get help.

- Difficulty feeding
- Difficulty putting on weight and retaining it
- Little interest in feeding
- Missing developmental milestones
- Difficulty making eye contact
- Poor muscle, eye or vision control
- Poor muscle tone
- Shaking hands or tremors
- Difficulty focusing or controlling impulses
- Walking on tiptoes
- Difficulty speaking
- Difficulty reading or spelling

WHAT TO DO IF YOUR CHILD IS SHOWING SIGNS OF HAVING ADDITIONAL CHALLENGES

The first thing you need to do is reach out to a health care professional – this could be your health visitor/public health nurse – or book an appointment with your doctor. Trust your mum gut and express your concerns. Sometimes you might have to press or fight for an answer, but you will know in your heart what needs to be done. The medical professionals will then start the process of running some standard tests and reports to help you get some answers as soon as they can – this can take some time and sometimes there isn't a definitive answer or diagnosis straight away and sometimes you may not even need a diagnosis. Your health care provider will help with all care and support whilst you navigate this journey. One thing is for sure: you won't be alone in this. There will be so many people out there wanting to love and support you.

Don't consult Dr Google, as tempting as this might be – this won't help, and you will jump to far too many conclusions. Speak with a medical professional who can help you and give you informed correct advice.

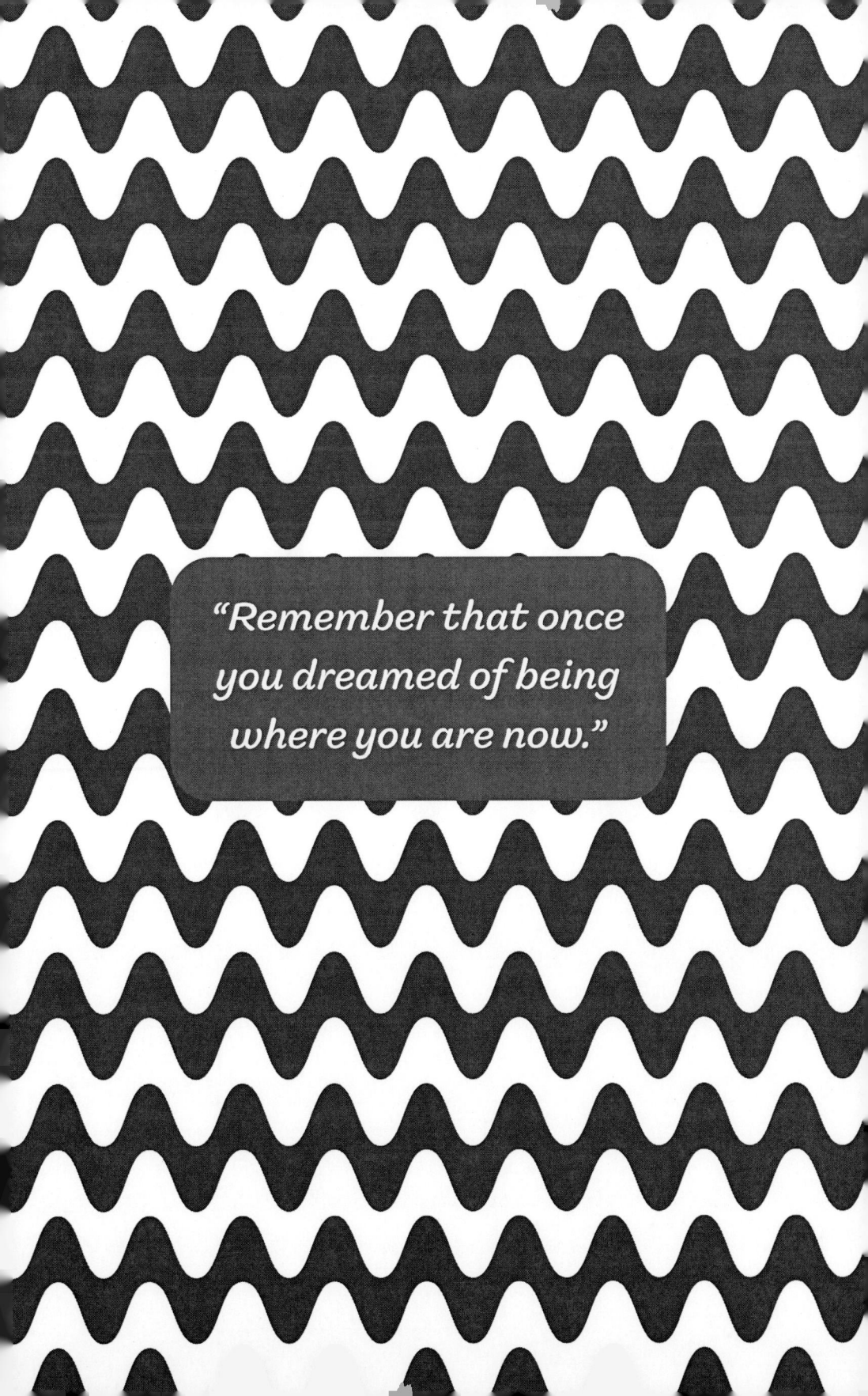

"Remember that once you dreamed of being where you are now."

Daily Journal

Date: _____

Daily Journal

Date: _____

Daily Journal

Date: _____

JOURNAL: WEEK FORTY-ONE

Daily Journal

Date: _____

Daily Journal

Date: _____

JOURNAL: WEEK FORTY-ONE

Daily Journal

Date: _____

Daily Journal

Date: _____

Weekly Check-In

Date: _____

Top 3 things I did this week:

_____

_____

_____

This week I felt:

Milestones:

Next week I would like to:

_____

_____

_____

Things I am proud of this week:

Things to celebrate:

Things to let go of:

My ranking of the week:

☆ ☆ ☆ ☆ ☆

JOURNAL: WEEK FORTY-ONE

Daily Journal

Date: _____

Daily Journal

Date: _____

Daily Journal

Date: _____

Daily Journal

Date: _____

Daily Journal

Date: _____

Daily Journal

Date: _____

Daily Journal

Date: _____

Weekly Check-In

Date: _____

Top 3 things I did this week:

_____

_____

_____

This week I felt:

Milestones:

Next week I would like to:

_____

_____

Things I am proud of this week:

Things to celebrate:

Things to let go of:

My ranking of the week:

☆ ☆ ☆ ☆ ☆

JOURNAL: WEEK FORTY-TWO

Daily Journal

Date: _____

Daily Journal

Date: _____

Daily Journal

Date: _____

Daily Journal

Date: _____

Daily Journal

Date: _____

Daily Journal

Date: _____

Daily Journal

Date: _____

Weekly Check-In

Date: _____

Top 3 things I did this week:

_____

_____

_____

This week I felt:

Milestones:

Next week I would like to:

_____

_____

_____

Things I am proud of this week:

Things to celebrate:

Things to let go of:

My ranking of the week:

☆ ☆ ☆ ☆ ☆

JOURNAL: WEEK FORTY-THREE

423

Daily Journal

Date: _____

_____
_____
_____
_____
_____
_____
_____
_____
_____
_____
_____
_____
_____
_____
_____
_____
_____
_____
_____
_____
_____
_____
_____
_____
_____
_____
_____
_____

Daily Journal

Date: _____

Daily Journal

Date: _____

Daily Journal

Date: _____

Daily Journal

Date: _____

Daily Journal

Date: _____

Daily Journal

Date: _____

JOURNAL: WEEK FORTY-FOUR

Weekly Check-In

Date: _____

Top 3 things I did this week:

_____

_____

_____

This week I felt:

Milestones:

Next week I would like to:

_____

_____

_____

Things I am proud of this week:

Things to celebrate:

Things to let go of:

My ranking of the week:

☆ ☆ ☆ ☆ ☆

JOURNAL: WEEK FORTY-FOUR   431

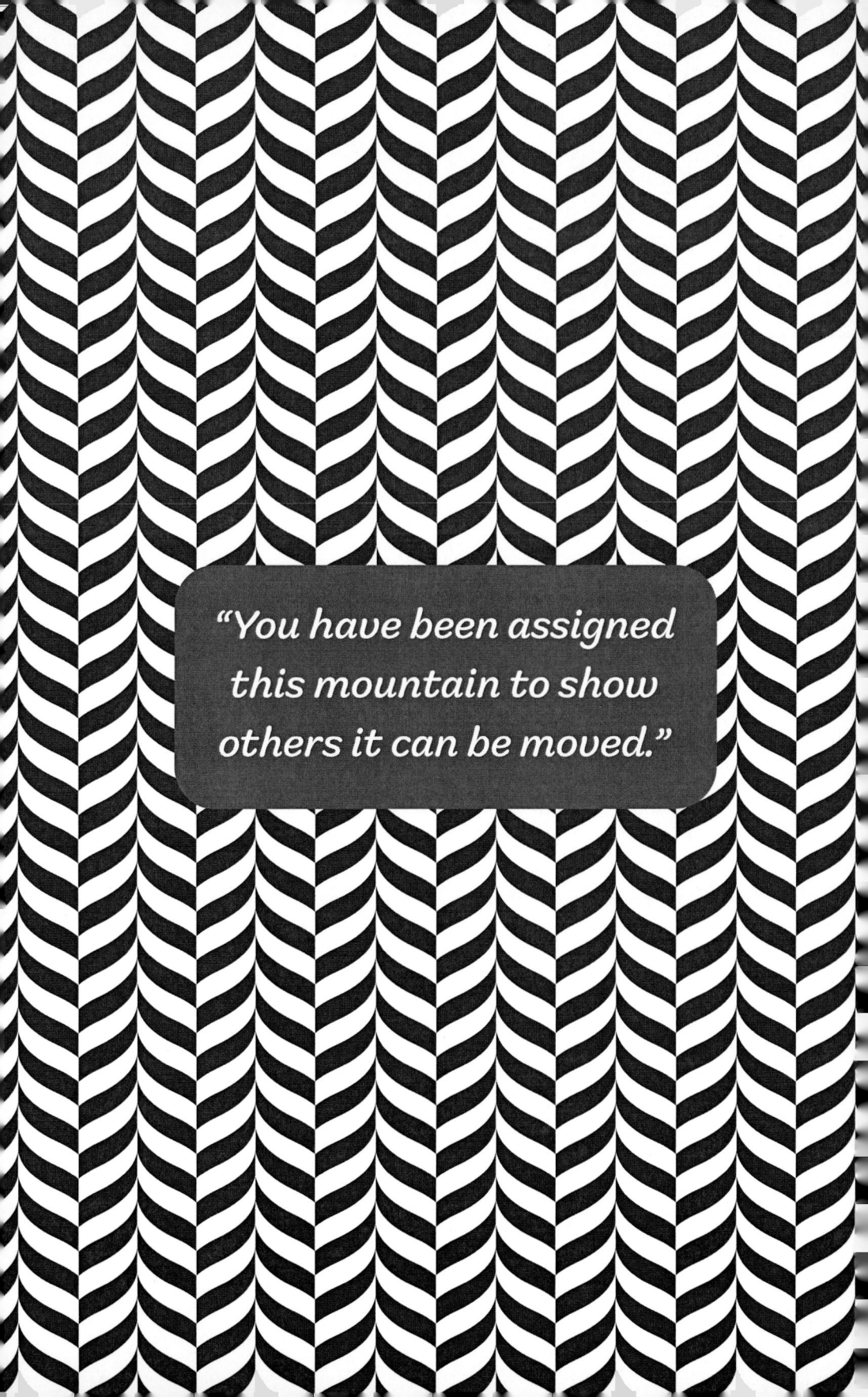

"You have been assigned this mountain to show others it can be moved."

POSITIVE ATTRIBUTES YOU WANT TO PASS ON TO YOUR CHILD

Picturing what you want to pass on to your children long-term can help you navigate how you want to parent them.

Often when you have your children, things from your own childhood can surface and come to light. They are highlighted and magnified massively. This can be a positive and healthy thing, as it can allow you to deal with past traumas or things you haven't accepted and allow you to work out what you would like to pass along and what you wouldn't pass along.

Your children more often than not look at who you are more than they listen to what you say. Writing down what attributes you want to pass on to them and then trying to model those attributes can make it much easier for them to follow suit.

> What you could include:
> - Your passion for something like creativity, music, a career
> - Importance of family and friend relationships
> - A grandparent's flair for gardening and working within nature
> - Your partner's humour
> - Self-resilience
> - How to put their mental health first
> - Kindness to themselves and others around them
> - A solid understanding of finances

Notes:

"Saying 'No' is okay."

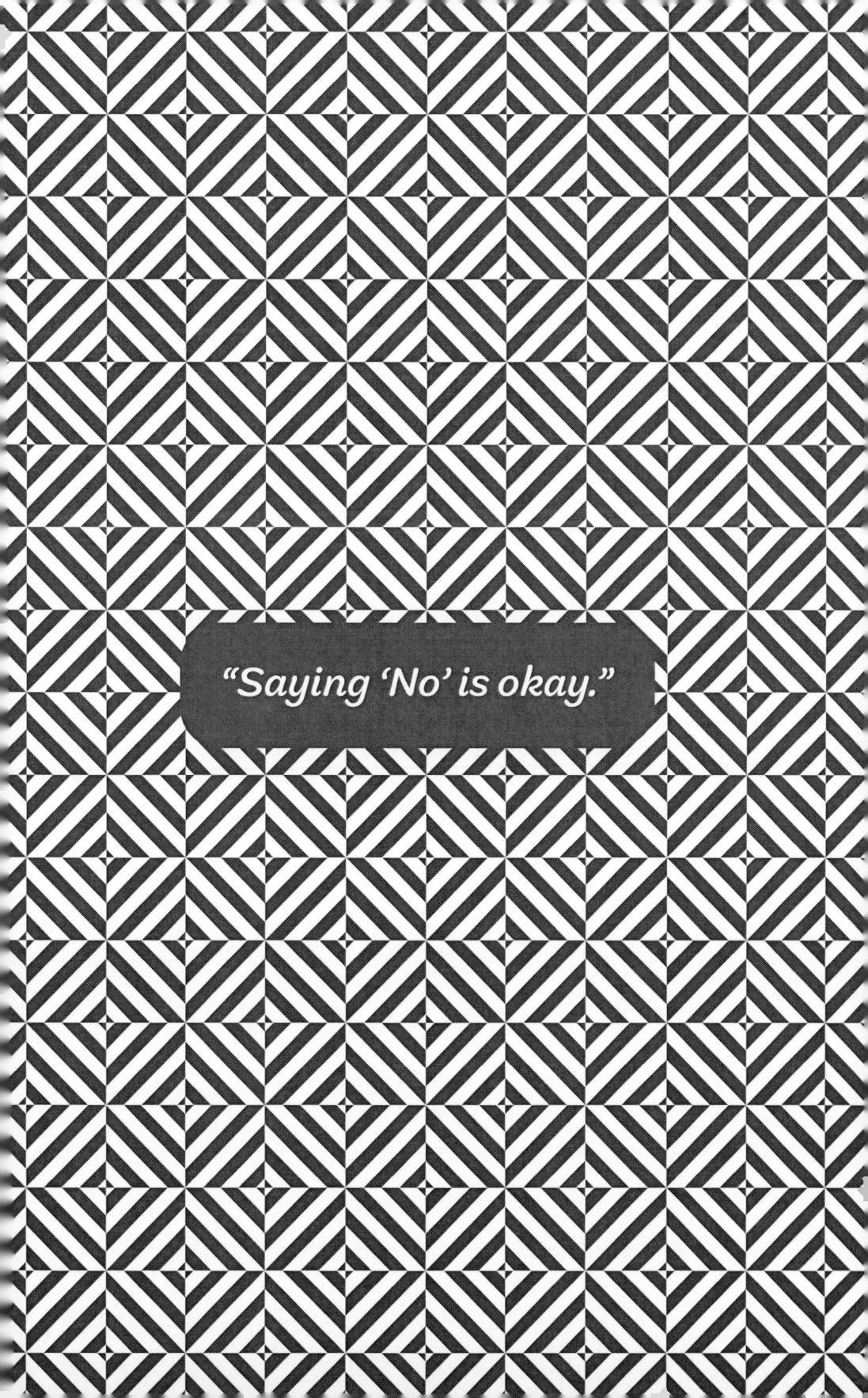

Daily Journal

Date: _____

Daily Journal

Date: _____

Daily Journal   Date: _____

Daily Journal

Date: _____

Daily Journal

Date: _____

Daily Journal

Date: _____

_____
_____
_____
_____
_____
_____
_____
_____
_____
_____
_____
_____
_____
_____
_____
_____
_____
_____
_____
_____
_____
_____
_____
_____
_____
_____

Daily Journal

Date: _____

Weekly Check-In

Date: _____

Top 3 things I did this week:

_____

_____

_____

Milestones:

This week I felt:

Next week I would like to:

_____

_____

_____

Things I am proud of this week:

Things to celebrate:

Things to let go of:

My ranking of the week:

JOURNAL: WEEK FORTY-FIVE

Daily Journal

Date: _____

JOURNAL: WEEK FORTY-SIX

Daily Journal

Date: _____

Daily Journal

Date: _____

Daily Journal

Date: _____

Daily Journal

Date: _____

Daily Journal

Date: _____

Daily Journal

Date: _____

Weekly Check-In

Date: _____

Top 3 things I did this week:

_____

_____

_____

Milestones:

This week I felt:

Next week I would like to:

_____

_____

_____

Things I am proud of this week:

Things to celebrate:

Things to let go of:

My ranking of the week:

☆ ☆ ☆ ☆ ☆

Daily Journal

Date: _____

Daily Journal

Date: _____

Daily Journal

Date: _____

Daily Journal

Date: _____

Daily Journal

Date: _____

Daily Journal

Date: _____

Daily Journal

Date: _____

Weekly Check-In

Date: _____

Top 3 things I did this week:

_____

_____

_____

This week I felt:

Milestones:

Next week I would like to:

_____

_____

_____

Things I am proud of this week:

Things to celebrate:

Things to let go of:

My ranking of the week:

☆ ☆ ☆ ☆ ☆

JOURNAL: WEEK FORTY-SEVEN

Daily Journal

Date: _____

Daily Journal

Date: _____

_____
_____
_____
_____
_____
_____
_____
_____
_____
_____
_____
_____
_____
_____
_____
_____
_____
_____
_____
_____
_____
_____
_____
_____
_____
_____
_____
_____

Daily Journal

Date: _____

JOURNAL: WEEK FORTY-EIGHT

Daily Journal

Date: _____

Daily Journal

Date: _____

Daily Journal

Date: _____

Daily Journal

Date: _____

JOURNAL: WEEK FORTY-EIGHT

Weekly Check-In

Date: _____

Top 3 things I did this week:

_____

_____

_____

Milestones:

This week I felt:

Next week I would like to:

_____

_____

_____

Things I am proud of this week:

Things to celebrate:

Things to let go of:

My ranking of the week:

☆ ☆ ☆ ☆ ☆

JOURNAL: WEEK FORTY-EIGHT 467

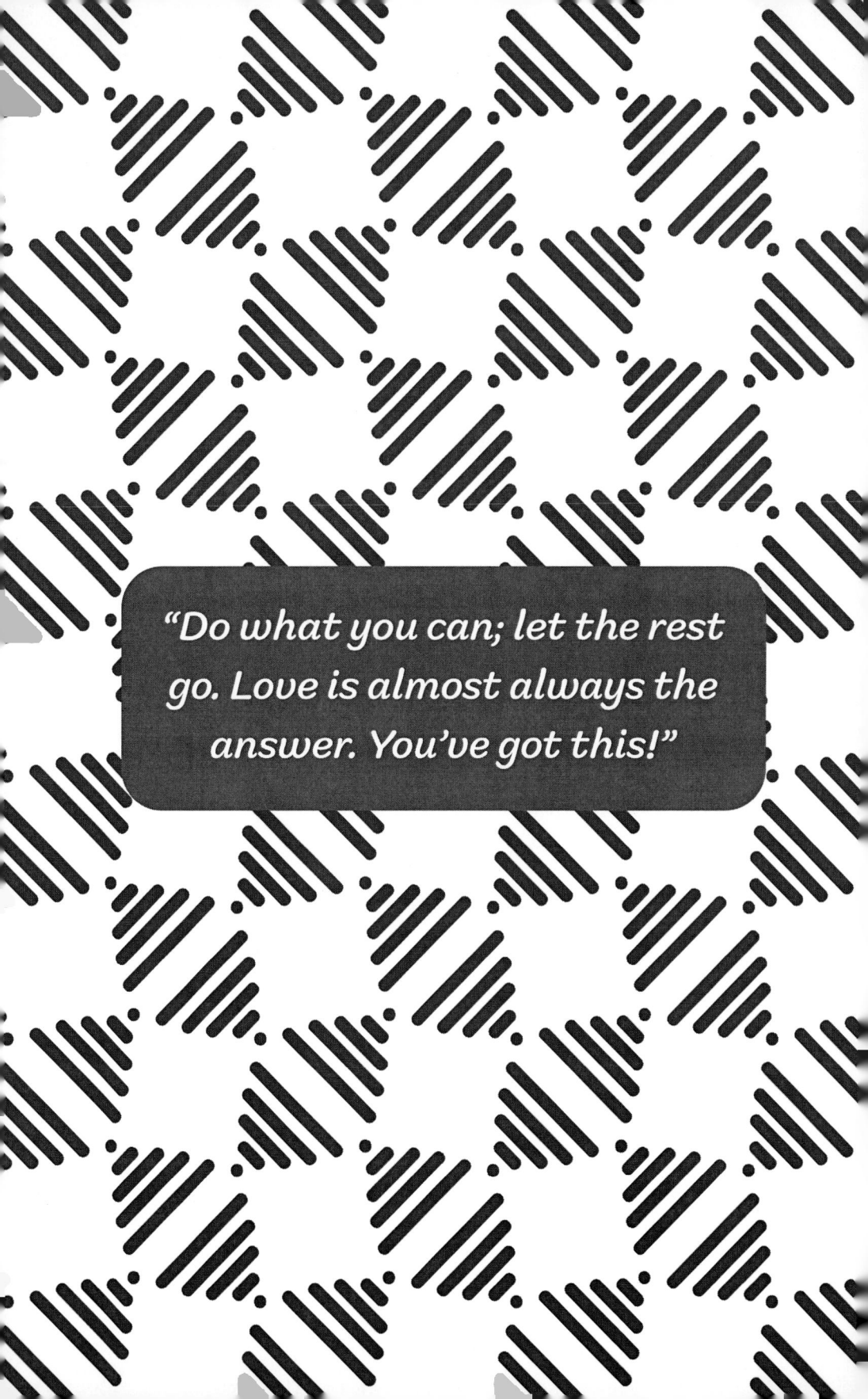

"Do what you can; let the rest go. Love is almost always the answer. You've got this!"

FUNNY STORIES FROM 'REAL LIFE MUMS'

Two memories that stand out... When Mollie was first out onto me, before we even knew what sex she was, she decided to greet me with a poo which went all down my side and body! Mollie used to always get hiccups, randomly at any time of day and night. It would scare the hell out of us during the middle of the night but it was a very sweet little noise from the Moses basket.

Amber – Mum of Mollie (3)

❋ ❋ ❋

Our dear friends popped over to announce that they were expecting their first baby, and they were very keen to help and get their practice in. During bath time, the baby ripped out a huge fart... started to do a wee... and I jumped into hyper-mum mode as I saw he was about to poop in the bath. I managed to catch 'some' of it in my hand... but the rest coated the whole bath. Safe to say, they left the room awkwardly laughing and didn't come back until it was all cleaned up and forgotten! Congratulations, guys!

Sarah – Mum of Cameron (2)

❋ ❋ ❋

When we had our second daughter, everything was going well until I caught our first born Eliza trying to put Poppy, who was six months at the time, in the office bin. I asked why and she said she 'didn't want a sister any more – it was too hard'!

Alice – Mum of Eliza (5) and Poppy (3)

❋ ❋ ❋

I remember researching EVERYTHING I possible could in the nine months that felt like forever waiting for Matilda to arrive. I had every gadget, resource and tool to help me on my journey into new motherhood and 'thought' I was super-prepared and knowledgeable. I bought a fancy steriliser that also dried the bottles, because who wants bottles that still have moisture on them? (Now have baby number two and realise this literally doesn't matter.) Anyway, I would take the bottles apart, pop them in the steriliser and for the first couple of days wondered what was wrong with it. I then realised after referring to my best friend Google, that you're supposed to wash them before putting them in to sterilise. Something which is now glaringly obvious was such a shock to my new-mum baby-brain! I thought my fancy new steriliser had failed to get them clean – we live and learn!

Margo – Mum of Matilda (3) and Delilah (6 months)

✼ ✼ ✼

I remember breastfeeding my son whilst trying to eat my dinner with the other hand and dropping food on his head! Oops!

Jess – Mum of Arlo (3) and Luna (10 months)

✼ ✼ ✼

The first time my husband changed Grayson's nappy in the hospital he weed all over him, he then got another nappy out and he did it again!!

Becca – Mum of Grayson (8 months)

✼ ✼ ✼

In the very early weeks, being constantly up at all hours of the night, I must have been changing my third or forth nappy of the night. Using my phone torch to make sure he was poo-free, I leant my face in to inspect his bum and at that moment Hugo farted and I felt a warm spray on my face. I couldn't help but laugh at how ludicrous life currently was. When breastfeeding there is always reason to cry over spilt milk. Breastfeeding Hugo on one boob and using a Hakka pump on the other, I had lost a morning sat on the sofa being milked like a cow. When Hugo was milk-drunk and the Hakka had collected a satisfying 4oz, it was time to escape. Without thinking, I stood up with baby in one hand and the Hakka pump gripped by my teeth, I swung my head forward to pull my hair back and the milk from the Hakka went all over my face, the baby and everything else that surrounded us.

Scarlett – Mum of Hugo (2)

✳ ✳ ✳

Seeing my husband's face (and managing to catch a photo of it) whilst he changed that first awful tar-filled nappy will never not be the funniest moment. The look of pure horror!

Courtney – Mum of Rafi (4 months)

✳ ✳ ✳

Jess had a rash when she was really little and someone said that breast milk was meant to be great for it. I sat for ages trying to get enough milk for her leg, I had about 15 mils, but as I wrangled my little one spilt it. So I resorted to hand squeezing my boob over her to get enough milk onto her rash… I really questioned my life choices in that moment – the rash didn't even clear up!!

Vikki – Mum of Jessica (2) and Emilia (3 months)

✳ ✳ ✳

My husband James would take Mason for his morning feed to give me a chance to catch up on sleep. He came in one morning going, 'Chloe, I need your help: Masons had an explosion.' I sleepily got out of bed and walked into his room to find he had pooed all over his nappy mat and on the curtain. I was not sure whether to be annoyed that I'd been woken up or impressed that he managed to poo on the curtain.

Chloe – Mum of Mason (1)

✳ ✳ ✳

I remember changing my son's nappy and halfway through he did the most explosive huge poo everywhere and then was sick. The worst thing was that the dog tried to get involved and trod poop down the hallway.

I didn't know if I should laugh or cry that we were both covered in all of the bodily fluids and now my dog and carpet were...

Rachel – Mum of Maddison (18 months)

***

I'd been away for a week with my three-month-old visiting family up North. My partner was so excited to see the baby when we got home, he held her up above his head, flying her around as it makes her laugh. Little did he realise I'd just fed her and regurgitated breast milk came right back up into his mouth!

Meg – Mum of Polly (7 months)

***

I was so sleep-deprived with my second born; we were going through sleep regression with both children and my brain had just given up. I took my littlest, who at the time was about three months old, to a class and I managed to forget her name... I still feel awful now!

Maddy – Mum of Thomas (4) and Daisy (1)

***

So first of all I had an awful labour which stretched over five days, so when my contractions finally came after the maximum amount of inductions I was like, 'Okay, any minute now'. It was 12 hours long, just this constant uncomfortable, moaning like a cow, all fours positioning. It was around hour eight, and the contractions were strong and about 90 seconds apart and all I could think was how much I hated my partner, like despised him, for not having to do anything but sit and wait. Mid-contraction, I was just like 'F**k this!' and I turned to him and said, 'If you wanted to extend our family a cat would've been easier.'

Lydia – Mum of Mila (3)

"Don't set yourself on fire to keep others warm."

Daily Journal

Date: _____

Daily Journal

Date: _____

Daily Journal

Date: _____

Daily Journal

Date: _____

Daily Journal

Date: _____

Daily Journal

Date: _____

Daily Journal

Date: _____

Weekly Check-In

Date: _____

Top 3 things I did this week:

_____

_____

_____

This week I felt:

Milestones:

Next week I would like to:

_____

_____

_____

Things I am proud of this week:

Things to celebrate:

Things to let go of:

My ranking of the week:

☆ ☆ ☆ ☆ ☆

JOURNAL: WEEK FORTY-NINE 481

Daily Journal

Date: _____

Daily Journal

Date: _____

Daily Journal

Date: _____

JOURNAL: WEEK FIFTY

Daily Journal

Date: _____

Daily Journal

Date: _____

Daily Journal

Date: _____

Daily Journal

Date: _____

Weekly Check-In

Date: _____

Top 3 things I did this week:

_____

_____

_____

This week I felt:

Milestones:

Next week I would like to:

_____

_____

_____

Things I am proud of this week:

Things to celebrate:

Things to let go of:

My ranking of the week:

JOURNAL: WEEK FIFTY

489

Daily Journal

Date: _____

Daily Journal

Date: _____

Daily Journal

Date: _____

Daily Journal

Date: _____

Daily Journal

Date: _____

Daily Journal

Date: _____

Daily Journal

Date: _____

Weekly Check-In

Date: _____

Top 3 things I did this week:

_____

_____

_____

This week I felt:

Next week I would like to:

_____

_____

_____

Things I am proud of this week:

My ranking of the week:

Milestones:

Things to celebrate:

Things to let go of:

JOURNAL: WEEK FIFTY-ONE

Daily Journal

Date: _____

Daily Journal

Date: _____

Daily Journal

Date: _____

JOURNAL: WEEK FIFTY-TWO

Daily Journal

Date: _____

Daily Journal

Date: _____

Daily Journal

Date: _____

Daily Journal

Date: _____

JOURNAL: WEEK FIFTY-TWO

Weekly Check-In

Date: _____

Top 3 things I did this week:

_____

_____

_____

Milestones:

This week I felt:

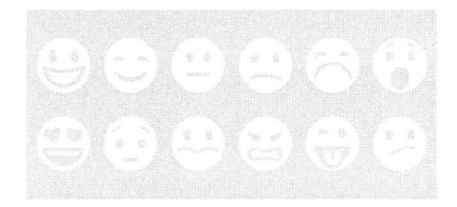

Next week I would like to:

_____

_____

_____

Things I am proud of this week:

Things to celebrate:

Things to let go of:

My ranking of the week:

☆ ☆ ☆ ☆ ☆

FILM & BOXSET RECOMMENDATIONS

BOXSETS

- Big Little Lies
- Working Morns
- Daisy Jones and the Six
- The Marvellous Mrs Maisel
- Firefly Lane
- The Night Agent
- Killing Eve
- Bridgerton
- Fleabag
- Citadel
- Friends
- Schitt's Creek
- The Big Bang Theory
- Breaking Bad
- Orange Is the New Black
- Good Girls
- Succession
- The Last of Us
- Gossip Girl
- Bad Sisters
- Outlander
- The Flight Attendant
- Big Little Lies
- The Good Wife
- Dead to Me
- Chuck
- Chicago Fire
- You
- And Just Like That
- SAS Rogue Heroes
- The Queen's Gambit
- Emily in Paris
- Happy Valley
- Desperate Housewives
- The Night Manager
- Normal People
- The Tourist
- Love Life
- Manifest
- Reacher
- The Buccaneers
- Shrinking
- The Morning Show
- The Continental
- Citadel

FILMS

- House of Versace
- Molly's Game
- Me Before You
- Legend
- Focus
- Bridesmaids
- The Holiday
- Life as We Know It
- The Greatest Showman
- Pretty Woman
- The Mother
- The Vow
- Extraction
- Queenpins
- The Hitman's Bodyguard
- Bad Moms 1 & 2
- Sex and the City
- Instant Family
- Notting Hill
- No Strings Attached
- Bridget Jones
- Knocked Up
- The Suicide Squad
- The Blind Side
- La La Land
- Hustlers
- Rush
- Say Yes
- I Don't Know How She Does It
- Mother's Day
- Gone Girl
- Cruel Intentions
- Bullet Train
- Persuasion
- The Great Gatsby
- Where the Crawdads Sing
- Heat
- Ghosted
- Dirty Dancing
- Britney Runs a Marathon
- Dumplin'
- Shotgun Wedding
- War Dogs
- Dog
- Crazy Rich Asians
- Gone Girl
- The Lost City
- The Covenant

"Focus on the step in front of you, not the whole staircase."
(Home Body Club)

Notes:

Notes:

Notes:

Notes:

Notes:

Notes:

"Worrying is like a rocking chair. It gives you something to do but it doesn't get you anywhere." (Erma Bombeck)